T0221110

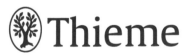

Training in Neurorehabilitation

Medical Training Therapy, Sports and Exercises

Sabine Lamprecht
Private Practice
Kirchheim
Germany

Hans Lamprecht
Private Practice
Kirchheim
Germany

158 illustrations

Thieme
Stuttgart • New York • Delhi • Rio de Janeiro

Library of Congress Cataloging-in-Publication Data is available from the publisher.

This book is an authorized translation of the 1st German edition published and copyrighted 2016 by Georg Thieme Verlag, Stuttgart. Title of the German edition: Training in der Neuroreha – Medizinische Trainingstherapie, Sport und Übungen

Translator: John Grossman, Schrepkow, Germany

Illustrator: Stefan Oldenburg, Heidelberg, Germany

© 2018 Georg Thieme Verlag KG

Thieme Publishers Stuttgart
Rüdigerstrasse 14, 70469 Stuttgart, Germany
+49 [0]711 8931 421, customerservice@thieme.de

Thieme Publishers New York
333 Seventh Avenue, New York, NY 10001, USA
+1 800 782 3488, customerservice@thieme.com

Thieme Publishers Delhi
A-12, Second Floor, Sector-2, Noida-201301
Uttar Pradesh, India
+91 120 45 566 00, customerservice@thieme.in

Thieme Publishers Rio, Thieme Publicações Ltda.
Edifício Rodolpho de Paoli, 25º andar
Av. Nilo Peçanha, 50 – Sala 2508
Rio de Janeiro 20020-906 Brasil
+55 21 3172 2297 / +55 21 3172 1896

Cover design: Thieme Publishing Group
Typesetting by DiTech Process Solutions Pvt. Ltd., India

Printed in Germany by CPI Books GmbH   5 4 3 2 1

ISBN 978-3-13-241585-0

Also available as an e-book:
eISBN 978-3-13-241586-7

Important note: Medicine is an ever-changing science undergoing continual development. Research and clinical experience are continually expanding our knowledge, in particular our knowledge of proper treatment and drug therapy. Insofar as this book mentions any dosage or application, readers mayrest assured that the authors, editors, and publishers have made every effort to ensure that such references are in accordance with **the state of knowledge at the time of production of the book.**

Nevertheless, this does not involve, imply, or express any guarantee or responsibility on the part of the publishers in respect to any dosage instructions and forms of applications stated in the book. **Every user is requested to examine carefully** the manufacturers' leaflets accompanying each drug and to check, if necessary in consultation with a physician or specialist, whether the dosage schedules mentioned therein or the contraindications stated by the manufacturers differ from the statements made in the present book. Such examination is particularly important with drugs that are either rarely used or have been newly released on the market. Every dosage schedule or every form of application used is entirely at the user's own risk and responsibility. The authors and publishers request every user to report to the publishers any discrepancies or inaccuracies noticed. If errors in this work are found after publication, errata will be posted at www.thieme.com on the product description page.

Some of the product names, patents, and registered designs referred to in this book are in fact registered trademarks or proprietary names even though specific reference to this fact is not always made in the text. Therefore, the appearance of a name without designation as proprietary is not to be construed as a representation by the publisher that it is in the public domain.

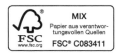

Contents

Preface... vi

1   Therapeutic Exercise 1
1.1   From Ancient Times to the Modern   1.3   From Orthopaedics to Neurology ..   4
      Age   1
1.2   From Bodybuilding to Medical
      Specialty..........................   3

2   Sports and Health 6
2.1   Significance of Movement........   6

3   General Effects of Training 11
3.1   Basic Motor Skills   11   3.5   Mobility   14
3.2   Strength   11   3.6   Coordination   16
3.3   Endurance   13   3.7   Balance   16
3.4   Speed.............................   13

4   Neurologic Rehabilitation 17
4.1   Cortical Reorganization   17   4.2   Feedback Training   30

5   Therapeutic Exercise in Neurology: Why?.................. 32
5.1   Introduction   32   5.3   Treatable Neurologic Symptoms
5.2   Factors Promoting Motor   in Therapeutic Exercise   34
      Learning   32

6   Training Equipment in Neurology 42
6.1   Training Equipment   42   6.6   Climbing...........................   71
6.2   Endurance Training   42   6.7   Small Devices for Training with
6.3   Strength Training   59   Neurologic Patients   72
6.4   Balance Training   63   6.8   Slacklining   72
6.5   Vibration Training   68   6.9   SilverFit..........................   72

7   Clinical Pictures.. 73
7.1   Introduction   73   7.7   Cerebral Palsy   87
7.2   Stroke   73   7.8   Neuromuscular Disorders   88
7.3   Multiple Sclerosis   78   7.9   Hereditary Spastic Paraplegia   95
7.4   Parkinson's Disease...............   81   7.10 Severely Impaired Patients and
7.5   Paraplegia   85   Therapeutic Exercise   95
7.6   Craniocerebral Trauma   86

8   Organizational Matters 96
8.1   Planning Training   96   8.3   Required Facilities   97
8.2   Personnel Requirements   97

9   Tests and Assessments 98
9.1   Tests for Neurorehabilitation   98

10   Further Reading 109

Preface

Neurorehabilitation constitutes an exciting area in the field of medical rehabilitation. For decades, therapeutic exercise has served as an integral part of musculoskeletal and cardiovascular rehabilitation. However, its significance as therapy for recovery from neurologic disorders has not been sufficiently explored. Why is it that therapeutic exercise has yet to become standard practice in the rehabilitation of neurologic patients?

Since the mid-1990s, we have been involved in the recovery of neurologic patients using therapeutic exercise regimens. Henceforth, we have been using the treadmill with body-weight-supported systems (BWST), strength and endurance training devices along with balance equipment, such as measuring platforms, mobile platforms, and the SpaceCurl, for a speedy recovery. Interestingly, even back then, many of these devices were computer controlled and equipped with feedback systems.

We began offering courses in therapeutic exercise in neurology in 2009. Since then, we continuously received requests for a book that could serve as a reference for the material covered in these courses.

There was no book that comprehensively examined the various aspects of therapeutic exercise and provided information on training for various neurologic disorders. However, recent times have witnessed a surge in the number of books and publications in professional journals dealing with specific diagnoses and aspects of appropriate therapy.

The notion that even people with neurologic disorders or symptoms can and should exercise is no longer as controversial as it was even a few decades ago. It is increasingly accepted that the main motor and functional problem in the neurologic patient is usually weakness. Thus, it is only natural to advise patients to exercise.

We have written this book in the hope of encouraging therapists to accompany their neurologic patients in the gym and have them participate in structured training programs developed according to the principles of therapeutic exercise.

We feel it is essential not to limit this planning to able-bodied neurologic patients, but also to include severely impaired patients (phase C). Our experience has shown that therapy often demands not too much, but too little, of neurologic patients, whether outpatient or inpatient.

We would particularly like to thank our neurologic patients, who — occasionally with some initial hesitation — have resolved to follow the arduous path of training to their tolerance limit and have come to realize that it is worth the effort. The positive and constructive feedback received from our patients has strengthened our resolve to document our findings in the form of this book.

It is our hope that the information provided here will assist physical therapists, occupational therapists, and sports therapists for the improvement and speedy recovery of their neurologic patients.

Sabine Lamprecht
Hans Lamprecht

1   Therapeutic Exercise

"To know what is good and not to put it into practice is tantamount to a lack of courage."

(Confucius)

1.1   From Ancient Times to the Modern Age

Even during ancient times, instructing patients on how to exercise on their own constituted a significant part of the therapy. Soranus of Ephesus (first to second century A.D.), whose lost manuscripts on acute and chronic diseases were preserved in the writings of the physician, Caelius Aurelianus (around 400 A.D.), declared that patients with paralysis should begin their first attempt at walking from a barber's chair (sella tonsoria). Later, they should practice walking using a sort of walker. To improve their steadiness, patients should be encouraged to practice on a sort of obstacle course incorporating various different ground surfaces and obstacles.[138]

The understanding of the relationship between movement and health passed from the Romans via Byzantium to Arab and Persian physicians. We are indebted to the Arab culture for having preserved the medical expertise of Greek and Roman physicians, which Arab scholars later expanded. Abu Ali Sina (c. 980–1037), known in Europe as Avicenna, wrote over 150 works and was one of the most renowned personalities of his age. A universal scholar, this Persian thinker explored physics, philosophy, astronomy, alchemy, and music in addition to medicine. His most famous work, "Qanun" (Canon medicinae) remained one of the most influential textbooks of medicine in Europe until into the 17th century.[138] Arab medicine was introduced into medieval Europe first and foremost by Jewish physicians from Spain and Portugal. Later, the medicine of the cloisters and monasteries influenced the field of medicine in central Europe during the Middle Ages. This monastic medicine regarded aiding the sick as a divine duty; the structured application of gymnastics or movement had no place in this philosophy of medicine. Only the renaissance in the 16th to 17th centuries ushered in a reevaluation of the positive effects on movement on health. In 1569, the Italian physician Hieronymus (Geronimo) Mercurialis (1530–1606) published his work,

"De Arte Gymnastica," in which he emphasized the importance of gymnastics for the preservation of health in ancient times.

Swedish poet and author Pehr Henrik Ling (1776–1839) is regarded as the inventor of Swedish Gymnastics and as one of the fathers of massage therapy. Ling travelled throughout Europe and took part in a naval battle; however, he suffered from rheumatism and experienced paralysis at a young age. Practicing fencing led to the improvement of his physical symptoms and eventually he was completely rehabilitated. In 1814, Ling founded the Central Gymnastics Institute in Stockholm and directed the institute until his death in 1839. The institute was later placed under the supervision of the ministry of education. While at the institute, he developed an entire system of precisely defined exercises as part of the gymnastics training program that needed to be performed in a highly specific sequence. Ling's "Swedish Gymnastics" influenced the history of physical therapy for many years.[364]

The Swedish physician Gustav Zander (1835–1920) is known for developing a system of exercise devices for physical therapy in the years after 1850. He invented medical mechanical therapy that was based on high-intensity physical training using mechanical force and movements to help people requiring medical gymnastics. His mechanistic approach to physical exercise came into existence with the establishment of Zander Institute, several of which were established throughout the world after 1870. Germany led the race with nearly 80 Zander Institutes. By 1905, the range of equipment included over 70 sophisticated exercise machines designed and built by Zander. He can rightly be called the proponent and inventor of the fitness studio and the franchise system. He was also a pioneer and trailblazer of today's equipment-based therapeutic exercise. The first government-certified training institution in Germany for physical therapy was established in the spring of 1901 as the Zander Institute; its director, Johann Hermann Lubinus, a Kiel physician, managed it as a medical mechanical institute.

Joseph Clément Tissot, a Swiss physician, described the early and timely rehabilitation of stroke patients based on structured physical therapy; however, it was not continued. On the contrary, the treatment for stroke recommended by the 1888 therapy guidelines of the Vienna General Hospital included this passage, "Apoplexia cerebri. Cerebral hemorrhage [...] furthermore a strict regime of bed rest, liquid nourishment. After about 2 months the residual paralyses are treated with faradization of the paralyzed extremities. Use of indifferent heat treatments. [...] Ensure regular bowel movements to prevent further strokes."[225]

Swiss physician Heinrich S. Frenkel (1860–1931) was one of the pioneers of neurologic rehabilitation. He introduced precise exercise instructions using specialized machines for the treatment of ataxia in tabes dorsalis and believed that only an intensive exercise regime integrated into the daily routine could lead to improved mobility and rapid recovery of patients. For instance, Frenkel, during an examination of a patient with tabes dorsalis, asked the patient to perform the finger-to-nose test. The patient performed poorly in the test; however, a few months later, the same patient returned and performed significantly better in the test. Frenkel could not understand the reason behind it. In response to Frenkel's query, the patient stated that he intended to perform well in the test the second time, he practiced the movement intensively. "The most important characteristic of the nervous substance is its ability to practice. This characteristic is based on the ability to reproduce in a peculiar way impressions or spoken very generally, states that have repeatedly and in the same manner taken hold of the nervous system."[132] Frenkel also noted that the mechanism of motor learning is not understood but that the "respective process often repeated itself." Furthermore, "to learn some new activity, three factors must work together: the perceived image of it, attentiveness, which places the image in the focus of consciousness and the repeated sequence of the activity."[132] Here Frenkel described the currently applicable concepts of motor learning and the possibilities of imagining movement.

Frenkel also understood the necessity of adapting exercises to the patient's level of performance, which we now refer to as "shaping." Frenkel equipped his room with various specialized training devices to improve his patients' dexterity and mobility by means of his special therapeutic gymnastics. His success was so profound that soon patients and an increasing number of physicians from all over Europe visited Frenkel in Heiden. F. Raymond, who succeeded J. M. Charcot as the chief of medical staff of the Hôpital Salpêtrière, sent R. Hirschberg, his assistant, to Heiden. Hirschberg was so impressed by Frenkel's treatment methods that he convinced Raymond and set up what was probably the first gymnasium in a neurologic clinic in the Hôpital Salpêtrière.[455] In 1896, Frenkel went to Berlin and worked at the Charité Hospital.

Otfrid Foerster (1873–1941), who spent two years with Frenkel in Heiden, intensively studied the neurology of motor activity. At the beginning of the 20th century, effective therapies in neurology hardly existed. Foerster published his ideas on motor rehabilitation in the form of manuals between 1916 and 1936, referring to them as "exercise therapy."[125,126] Also, he developed a guideline for treating central palsies.[139]

In the early 20th century, facilities for patients with posttraumatic conditions were established, as were "cripple homes" for children with birth trauma or congenital deformities. Until then patients in the chronic stage were not considered eligible and therefore, did not receive any support from the statutory health insurance fund and were primarily dependent on the municipal aid to the poor.[288] In 1907 orthopaedist K. Biesalski called for the establishment of a public "cripple care program" with the slogan, "turn charity recipients into taxpayers."

In 1909, the German Association for Cripple Care was founded, the forerunner of the present-day German Association for Rehabilitation. Between 1906 and 1914, the Oskar Helene Home was built with the financial support of industrialists, Oskar and Helene Pintsch, to care for children and adolescents with orthopaedic and neurologic disabilities. This home is regarded as the first rehabilitation clinic in Germany.[138] Children and adolescents in the Oskar Helene Home received medical care, attended the school affiliated with the home, and were provided the opportunity to learn a trade in its specially developed workshops. The excellent outcomes of this rehabilitation led to the unanimous passing of the Prussian Cripple Care Act in 1920 by the Prussian legislature, with Biesalski playing an instrumental role in formulating the bill. This was the first time that an entitlement to medical care and occupational integration became law.[288] Until his death in 1930, Biesalski managed the Oskar Helene Home in Berlin together with Hans Schütz (1875–1958), an influential proponent of "cripple education." In 1934, the home was placed under the control of Hitler's SS squadron ("Schutzstaffel"). Henceforth, the senior physicians at Oskar Helene Home aided in implementing the Law on the Prevention of Progeny with Hereditary Disease.[288]

World War I provided a new impetus for neurorehabilitation, as specialized military hospitals and rehabilitation facilities were set up for wounded servicemen. The large number of soldiers suffering brain injuries (250,000–300,000) in World War I necessitated the establishment of specialized facilities, one of them being the introduction of the steel helmet. The Frankfurt Institute for Brain Trauma Patients headed by Kurt Goldstein (1878-1965) held a preeminent position in terms of both therapy and scientific research. The head of the psychological institute was Adrémar Gelb (1887-1936). The two men jointly authored numerous publications on the behavior of individuals with brain trauma.[138] These military hospitals for brain trauma patients combined purely surgically oriented treatment with recovery based on psychological and occupational rehabilitation.

The advancements achieved in the field of neuro and psychotherapy suffered a major setback during the Nazi period. The era witnessed the abandonment of many of the research approaches for the rehabilitation of neurologic patients, forcing several prominent neurologists to emigrate. In 1942, leading neurologists ensured that psychologists were prohibited from working in the special military hospitals for soldiers with brain injuries.[138] The history of neurorehabilitation after World War II is also a story of forced emigration, as many leading specialists, including Goldstein, Gelb, Isserlin, and Fröschel, were compelled to leave Germany.[138]

Friedrich Schmieder (1911–1988) is regarded as one of the pioneers of modern neurologic rehabilitation in postwar Germany. In November 1950, Schmieder founded the Sanatorium Schloss Rheinburg in Gailingen am Hochrhein that was initially equipped with 20 beds for private patients with neurologic and psychiatric disorders. A legal entitlement to rehabilitation was introduced in 1957, and in 1960, the sanatorium in Gailingen was transformed into a specialized neurologic clinic. Currently, the Schmieder Clinic includes six neurologic and rehabilitation clinics in the German state of Baden-Württemberg and covered all phases of neurologic rehabilitation.

From the beginning, Schmieder propagated the concept of brain training in his clinics. He felt that the holistic treatment of neurophysiologic ("physical") and neurocognitive ("mental") symptoms including intensive psychotherapeutic care was crucial to optimally improve and promote the quality of life of his patients and their social participation. In 1956, he elucidated his holistic approach to the treatment of neurologic and psychiatric disorders in a memorandum to the German minister of labor:

"Should the therapeutic process partially restore or exercise physical and mental capabilities, then it still may not necessarily have achieved what must be the focal point of rehabilitation. We mean the knowledge of one's remaining capabilities and opportunities for development, regaining hope and the courage to face life, ascertaining one's future social and occupational path, and especially the readiness to integrate into the social world and assume a certain risk in life."[359]

Schmieder's five principles dovetail perfectly with the basic principles of today's therapeutic exercise in neurology:

- Lifelong learners achieve better results, in other words, those who train lifelong achieve longer.
- Writing down means remembering better.
- Training includes exercise and breaks.
- Movement helps the brain perform better.
- Training the brain mobilizes the brain reserves, in other words, training mobilizes the brain's reserves.

1.2 From Bodybuilding to Medical Specialty

The popular American Vaudeville shows transformed muscles and strength into attractions through stage acts and performances in the late 19th century. These acts included skilled dancers, musicians, actors, comedians, magicians, trained animals, and athletes. Eugene Sandow (stage name), one of the proponents of weightlifting, was born in 1867 in Königsberg, Germany, as Friedrich Wilhelm Müller. From 1896 onward, he started touring the United States with various traveling shows, especially performing strongman stunts such as lifting a horse. A born performer, he soon popularized weightlifting in the United States, eventually spreading it throughout the country. Sandow capitalized on his appearance and held the first bodybuilding competition in London in 1901. This competition is regarded as the forerunner to the international Mr. Olympia competition of the International Federation of Bodybuilding and Fitness introduced by Joe Weider in 1965. Austrian-born Arnold Schwarzenegger was the world's most successful bodybuilder in the 1960s and 1970s. In the wake of Schwarzenegger's initial Hollywood success, bodybuilding experienced an increasing boom in Europe, especially in the years following 1982.

The concept of strength training in fitness studios gradually gave rise to the idea of applying the findings of scientific sports research to the rehabilitation of individuals suffering from musculoskeletal disorders. The Norwegian physiotherapist, Oddvar Holten, published the article "Medisinsk Treningsterapie" in the professional journal, "Fysioterapeuten" in 1962 that focused on medical training therapy. In treating athletes, he found that the athletes showed a greater and sustained improvement of symptoms if their manual treatment or therapy was integrated into suitably adapted active exercises (exercise therapy) and termed it as "grading the exercise." His efforts led the Norwegian Ministry of Health to recognize therapeutic exercise as a form of therapy as early as 1967. This was followed by the introduction of therapeutic exercise in Germany as a "specially indicated therapy" by the Administrative Employers' Liability Insurance Association in 1983. Currently, therapeutic exercise is the mainstay of rehabilitation in musculoskeletal disorders (▶ Fig. 1.1).

Cardiovascular rehabilitation, especially after a heart attack, has also undergone a paradigm shift in the last 30 years. Patients who have suffered a heart attack must take special care by involving themselves in specific training to strengthen their cardiac systems to prevent any future events. In this regard, therapeutic exercise has become an integral part of the rehabilitation of patients with

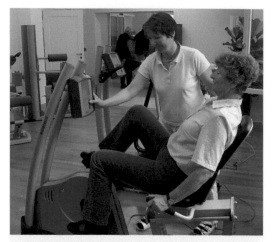

Fig. 1.2 Ergometer training.

cardiovascular disorders. For this reason, equipment, such as ergometers and other endurance devices, constitute an essential part of the rehabilitation process of these patients (▶ Fig. 1.2).

1.3 From Orthopaedics to Neurology

The realization that motor learning in patients with neurologic deficits is no different than in normal individuals means that the same principles of training in surgical and orthopaedic rehabilitation can be applied to neurologic rehabilitation. In the early 1990s, Hesse et al[173] studied the effects of treadmill therapy with body weight–support systems in poststroke patients and demonstrated its efficacy (▶ Fig. 1.3).

In recent years, the success of training has been demonstrated with many neurologic disorders. However, this knowledge has been slow to find ts way into the daily routine of neurologic rehabilitation. Many new findings in neurologic rehabilitation are based on the understanding of motor learning. These findings come from scientific studies in training and sports research.

Examples include:

- **Repetitive exercise:** Repetitions improve the motor outcomes in terms of both quality and quantity.
- **Mental practice:** Long practices in sports and occupational settings are yet to gain widespread acceptance in neurologic rehabilitation.

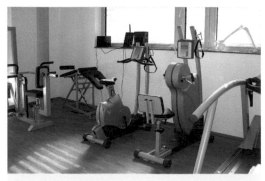

Fig. 1.1 Exercise room.

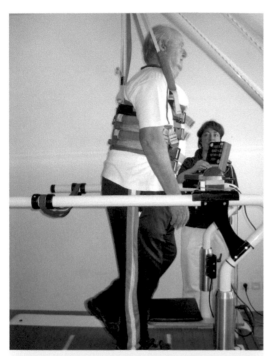

Fig. 1.3 Treadmill with body weight–support system.

Many other fundamentals of motor learning used in the training of athletes may also be found in identical or similar forms in the new approaches in neurologic rehabilitation.

The future and the daily routine of therapists in neurologic rehabilitation are changing. The introduction of new devices in neurorehabilitation is an inexorable process. Physical therapists and occupational therapists must address this new challenge so that the knowledge and experience of these occupational groups continue to contribute to rehabilitation. If these two occupational groups are unwilling to face this challenge, they will eventually be replaced by well-trained sports scientists. Unfortunately, the time required for the findings of scientific therapy research to get accepted and incorporated into the daily routine of inpatient facilities is relatively long. Usually, a considerable time lapses before these findings are reflected in outpatient practice. Yet, it takes much longer for healthcare providers to incorporate these findings into the framework agreements or include them in the range of health-care services.

It has been known since the late 19th century that the nervous system has the capability to adapt its own structures and functions in response to new challenges. The use of rapidly evolving imaging modalities with increasingly high resolution has provided us with detailed and enhanced understanding of the plasticity of the nervous system. Studies suggest that functional reorganization of the motor cortex occurs both as a result of a lesion in the central or peripheral nervous system (lesion-induced plasticity) and as a consequence of motor training (training-induced plasticity).[111,384] Mulder[277] refers to humans in this context as "congenital adapters."

2 Sports and Health

"Whoever does not do something for his health every day will one day have to sacrifice very much time for his illness."

(Sebastian Kneipp)

2.1 Significance of Movement

"There is no medication that has as many desirable effects and as few side effects as movement. Movement as a medication has one big disadvantage! It must be actively produced by the patient himself with some effort." (Paul Haber according to Mayr et al.[257])

For over 10,000 years, the human body has been attuned to delivering high performance on demand (▶Fig. 2.1). With rapid industrialization, our living and working conditions have changed radically. Nevertheless, neither the human metabolism nor musculature underwent drastic changes during these times. Moreover, physical exertion is a rare aspect for the majority of people belonging to the economically well-developed societies. Consequently, a sedentary lifestyle and improper nutrition are among the greatest problems faced by these industrialized societies. The consequences

are well known and include high blood pressure, diabetes, arteriosclerosis, stroke, depression, obesity, cancer, and back problems (▶Fig. 2.2).

We cannot deny or reverse evolution. For thousands of years, humans were dependent on hunting, working, or walking for their food and livelihood, implying that humans tended to be on a constant move the whole day. For instance, the cavemen of the Stone Age had a radius of movement of about 40 kilometers (25 miles). It is intriguing that despite the involvement in vigorous physical activities, the biology of human body has not undergone much change since the Stone Age. However, as industrialization has progressed, the amount of physical work we perform has steadily decreased resulting in a considerable stationary lifestyle (▶Fig. 2.3).

The modernization and urbanization has bestowed on the human society countless facilities encouraging reduced physical labor. The lack of

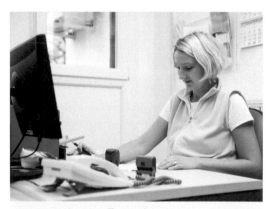

Fig. 2.2 Sedentary office work.

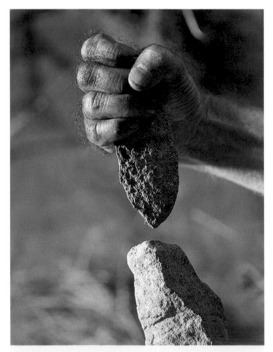

Fig. 2.1 Caveman in the Stone Age.

Note

Because of our current inactive lifestyle, primarily a result of industrialization, we often hardly engage ourselves in physical activities requiring robust body movement; if at all, the movement is light to moderate. This has led to the familiar diseases of modern civilization related to reduced activity, such as obesity and cardiovascular disorders, which can largely be avoided by involving oneself in activities requiring sufficient movement.

physical activity and movement initiates at a very early stage, for instance, with schoolchildren who no longer walk to school. Cooper et al[67] demonstrated that children who walk to school are physically more active and fit even after school hours as compared to the children who ride to school in a car. (▶ Fig. 2.4)

The question whether the daily physical performance of children and adolescents has undergone substantial change over the last few years and

decades is the basis of a study by Bös.[43] Bös included international studies between 1965 and 2002 and compared the results of five test tasks in four age groups, which were divided by gender into four study cohorts (until 1997, 1976–1985, 1986–1995, and after 1996). The results demonstrated a significant worsening of the measured achievements in four of the five test tasks (▶ Fig. 2.5).[43] In persons with a low level of physical activity, the number of inflammatory factors, especially interleukin-6 (IL-6) and tumor necrosis factor alpha (TNF-α), detectable in the bloodstream, was significantly lower than in physically active individuals. These immune system–activating molecules are continuously secreted by enlarged fat cells and contribute to the development and progression of diseases afflicting the modern civilization.

It has never been completely explained why athletic activity exerts a positive influence on these factors. For example, blood IL-6 is increased by a factor of up to 100 after an athletic activity. Yet, IL-6, like TNF-α and interleukin-1 (IL-1), is among the first messenger-α substances that are excreted during an inflammation by the immune cells. This, in turn, activates an entire cascade of other inflammatory molecules that are then detectable in the bloodstream.

Under normal physiological circumstances, inflammatory substances do not circulate in the blood (▶ Fig. 2.6). These inflammatory substances are normally excreted by the body to combat pathogens, remove damaged tissue, or stimulate healing processes. However, in physically inactive or older individuals, the level of these inflammatory substances in the blood is often permanently

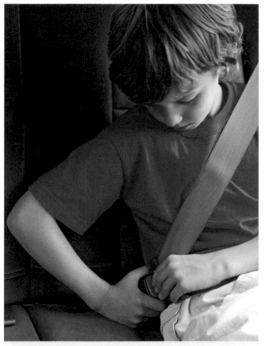

Fig. 2.3 Car passenger.

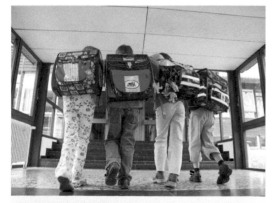

Fig. 2.4 Schoolchildren.

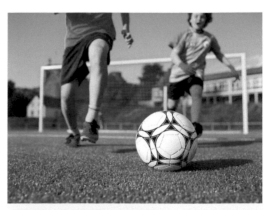

Fig. 2.5 Children practicing sports.

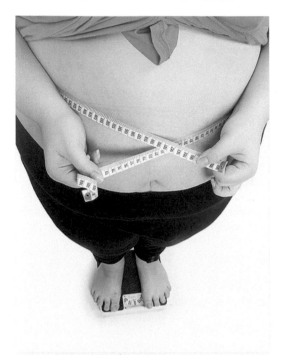

Fig. 2.6 Obesity.

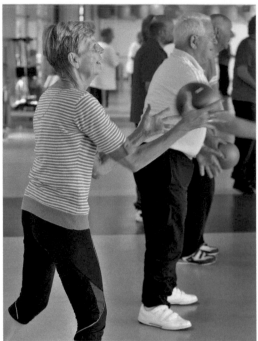

Fig. 2.7 Sports in old age.

elevated. The body is thus constantly in a defensive state with a low-grade inflammation. In contrast, far fewer of these inflammatory substances are found in the bloodstream of physically active people. It can be said that the fitter a person is, the fewer messenger molecules will circulate in that person's bloodstream.

Scientists report that during physical activity, the musculature excretes chemicals known as myokines.[298] Nearly 400 chemical substances are produced by the skeletal muscles during various physical activities; however, the mode of action of only about a dozen is understood. Considering the fact that musculature is one of the body's largest organs, the effects of these myokines should not be underestimated. These chemicals function in the most complex manner. For instance, it is not yet completely understood why the secretion of IL-6, whose concentration in the blood is increased by a factor of up to 100 during sports, should have a calming effect on the defensive state of human body. Pedersen advanced the theory that during sports activity, the level of IL-6 increases sharply, whereas the level of TNF drops. Handschin[162] feels that the rapid excretion of IL-6 triggers an immediate responsive reaction by the body, finally leading

to the excretion of interleukin-10 (IL-10), which, in turn, attenuates the effect of the defensive immune reaction.

These proposed explanations support the notion that even patients with chronic inflammatory processes such as rheumatoid arthritis should actively participate in sports to positively influence their physical constitution. However, these myokines appear to have multiple functions in the human body apart from influencing the inflammatory substances in the blood. These include regulation of fat metabolism, influencing the blood vessels, and assisting the function of the liver. It is also thought that the myokines have an effect on the brain and help protect against dementia.[298]

> ### Note
>
> It is never too late to develop athletic activities to benefit from the positive effects of sports and movement. The effectiveness of training has been scientifically proven even for 90-year-olds and persons with chronic diseases (▶ Fig. 2.7).[456]

A 2005 publication by the German Ministry of Health studied the number of steps taken by certain selected occupational groups during their daily work. It was found that several working people could not reach the recommended daily number of steps. The study found that the participants averaged 3,000 steps (about 2.4 km or 1.5 miles). However, the optimum degree of movement is around 10,000 steps per day, meaning an individual should walk about 8 km or 5 miles every day. Therefore, to even approach this goal, the basic recommendation for everyone is to increase their locomotion activity in daily life. Whenever possible, walking should be preferred to driving, and the use of stairs to using the elevator (▸ Fig. 2.8). Moreover, everyone can determine their individual number of steps using a pedometer.

Various studies recommend physical activity so that people can benefit from the positive effects.[165,294,290] Thirty minutes of moderate activity 5 days a week (150 minutes per week) is regarded as the minimum. Yet, another study demonstrated that even 15 minutes of activity per day has a positive impact on health.[427]

Various epidemiologic studies suggest that an able-bodied untrained adult must figure on decreased performance and an increased risk of disease if certain patterns of muscle use are no longer regularly applied (▸ Fig. 2.9).

The positive effects of sports and movement have been clearly demonstrated. The most important points include:

- Sports and sufficient movement reduce weight.
- The cholesterol level is reduced or normalized.
- The risk of contracting osteoporosis is reduced.
- Both systolic and diastolic blood pressure values are reduced.
- The insulin level is reduced and the blood glucose level normalized.
- The risk of cancer is reduced.
- Arteriosclerosis is less likely to develop.
- The risk of developing depression is reduced (▸ Fig. 2.10).

These important positive effects naturally apply to persons with neurologic deficits as well. Neurologic patients are often limited in their mobility owing to their neurologic symptoms. Therefore, guidance and encouragement to practice sports are important so that patients can benefit from the positive effects of these activities.

Sports and movement also offer these patients a good opportunity for social interaction with a group of like-minded people (▸ Fig. 2.11).

> **Note**
>
> Failure to tense every skeletal muscle with at least 30% of maximum strength at least once a day and exert the cardiovascular system to at least 50% of maximum capacity for more than 5 minutes a day is associated with decreased performance and increased risk of morbidity.[198]

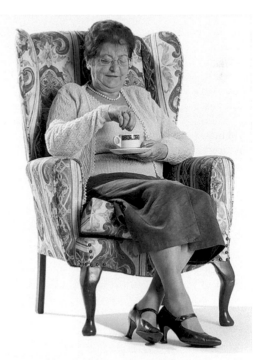

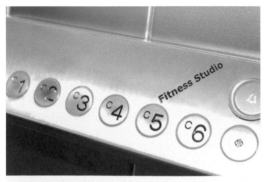

Fig. 2.8 Taking the elevator to the fitness studio.

Fig. 2.9 Whoever rests, rusts.

Therefore, all patients and neurologic patients in particular, should be provided guidance and encouraged to move around in their daily lives and participate in sport activities. Trained therapists with neurologic experience must be available as coaches and contacts for these patients in various facilities, such as sports clubs, fitness studios, and therapeutic exercise facilities, so that these patients can engage in sports in accordance with their needs and abilities.

Back in 1875 the internist Oertel offered physical training to patients with various heart disorders (Terrain therapy, ▶Fig. 2.12).[185] In contrast to the predominant medical consensus at the time, which recommended bed rest and passive treatment applications, Oertel prescribed gymnastic exercises to his patients and suggested they go hiking. He was highly successful with this. However, these findings sank into oblivion. It was only after World War II that interest in these activities was revived.

Today sports and physical training are considered as the standard for many patients undergoing rehabilitation. Sports are no longer regarded as a taboo even for neurologic patients. Patients are now recommended to regularly keep moving. Which sport should be recommended for a particular severity of disease is naturally a question that must be decided on an individual basis.

Note

Neurologic disorders and sports activities are not mutually exclusive. Sports participation also exert therapeutic effects on neurologic patients (▶Fig. 2.13).

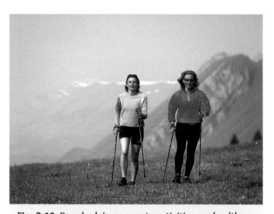

Fig. 2.10 Regular leisure sports activities are healthy.

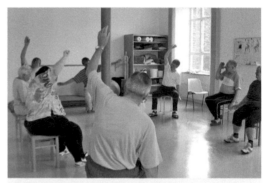

Fig. 2.11 Parkinson group.

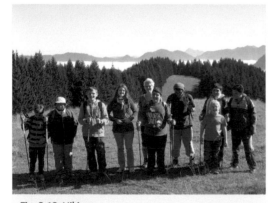

Fig. 2.12 Hiking.

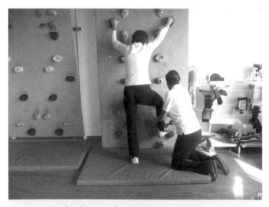

Fig. 2.13 Climbing with patients with multiple sclerosis.

3 General Effects of Training

"What is beautiful in all things is the proper mean. I do not like excess and deficiency."

(Democritus)

3.1 Basic Motor Skills

Training is an integral part of our life and involves adapting the body to physical activity. We train our muscles every time we move. Sports researchers have studied the effects of training in able-bodied people and athletes for many years and have published a wealth of scientific findings. Inactivity leads to a rapid loss of strength and muscular endurance in healthy musculature and is associated with muscle fiber atrophy. A simultaneous derangement of mitochondrial function occurs with a reduction in the activity of oxidative enzymes. This is known as the deconditioning syndrome. Deconditioning syndrome occurs especially in posttraumatic and postoperative situations or in chronic disorders.

A decrease in the physical performance results in a decreased exercise tolerance. This leads to a situation in which even slight exertion can produce symptoms of overload. This means that the patient avoids the exertion, which in turn, exacerbates the deconditioning syndrome, thereby creating a vicious circle, which must be broken.

There is no pharmaceutical alternative to training to improve performance. The goal of training is to improve or restore performance. This is referred to as reconditioning.

Inactivity leads to a general reduction in physical performance and activity in both healthy and sick individuals. Many patients exhibit an increased inactivity for a variety of reasons. This means it would be important, particularly for patients with chronic disorders, to train. In spite of this, many neurologic patients are still instructed to relax. Yet, this is counterproductive, as it exacerbates the deconditioning syndrome.

Training is the effort to act on the body by means of targeted measures with the goal of improving or maintaining performance. In a rehabilitation setting, this goal is to eliminate performance deficits and bring about an improvement in performance. Therefore, training can improve a person's performance in general as well as tuning his/her neuromuscular coordination. Training can also be used to learn motion sequences and gradually optimize them.

▶ Basic motor skills include:
- Strength
- Endurance
- Speed
- Coordination
- Balance
- Mobility

3.2 Strength

The term "strength" refers to different skills. These different skills can be regarded separately. However, it should be clearly understood that these skills never occur in isolation in daily life (▶ Fig. 3.1).

Muscular strength is measured with the Medical Research Council scale (▶ Table 5.4).

▶ Medical Research Council (MRC) Scale of Muscular Strength.
0 No muscular activity, complete paralysis
1 Visible and/or palpable contraction without movement
2 Movement is possible when gravity is neutralized
3 Movement against gravity is just barely possible
4 Movement against slight resistance
5 Normal strength

Definition [ ]

Strength is defined as the capability of the neuromuscular system to perform concentric, eccentric, or static work by means of contraction. This occurs as a result of innervation and metabolic processes.

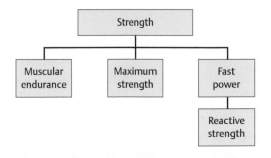

Fig. 3.1 Strength and strength skills.

Strength training involves placing a mechanical load on the muscle. This leads to an increase in the myofibril proteins, whereas the mitochondria and capillaries remain largely unchanged.[188] Rapid neuromuscular adaptation occurs at the beginning of strength training; neural activity is increased and the synchronization of the motor units is improved. Activation of a larger number of motor units combined with the simultaneous reduction in antagonist coactivity leads to rapid improvement of strength. Muscle hypertrophy occurs only when strength training is continued over a period of weeks and months.[134]

3.2.1 Strength Training in Neurologic Rehabilitation

Strength training is essential for neurologic rehabilitation; yet, it has little in common with body building. The goal is not to increase muscle mass but to improve overall strength to enable normal daily functions and activities. This view will lead to a paradigm shift in neurologic rehabilitation.

Many traditional physical therapy concepts have clearly opposed strength training in the past and some still do. This thinking reflects a number of reservations, for example, strength training might exacerbate spasticity or the assumption that the function itself is present but the patient does not yet have access to it. Critics thus concluded that strength training in neurology is at best unnecessary and may even be harmful to the patient. Many therapists are of the opinion that a neurologic patient does not feel the movement and as a result cannot perform it, making sensitivity training far more useful and effective than strength training.

It is safe to conclude that the subject of strength or loss of strength has been seriously neglected in neurologic rehabilitation. The effects are still felt today because these views are often propagated further without reflection. Unfortunately, this is also the case in the training of physical therapists at certain physical therapy schools.

Even the guidelines of the German Society of Neurologic Rehabilitation (DGNR)[312] refer to the importance of strength training in treatment of the arm as a class B recommendation. Class B means that the recommendation is advisable as opposed to mandatory and is based on well-designed clinical studies, albeit not randomized studies.

Training muscular endurance and power is crucial in neurologic rehabilitation. Examples of important focal points of strength training in neurologic patients include proximal strength deficits in the

shoulder girdle leading to difficulties in lifting the arm and strength deficits in the knee extensors leading to difficulties in performing a functional knee extension. Eickhof published a study in 2001 in which she centered her therapy on the issue of upper extremity palsy in patients (Chapter 4).[108]

The quadriceps constitute an important group of muscles for the function of the lower extremity, particularly, walking. Weakness in the quadriceps leads to hyperextension of the knee (Physiolexikon).[306] As the leg is unable to support the full weight of the body in functional extension, the body compensates by locking the knee in hyperextension. This provides the patients a strategy for holding their full body weight on one leg in the stance phase. However, an 80-kg (176-lb) patient must be able to move at least his weight both concentrically and eccentrically several times with one leg.

It has often been stated that the quadriceps in neurologic patients are considerably strong. However, testing is not performed with an 80-kg weight but with far less weight in easy positions, such as with both legs. There are also various gait analyses that have found minimal quadriceps activity in the walking patient. It is important to note that these analyses were performed in able-bodied subjects at a normal walking pace of about 120 steps per minute. However, the walking pace in neurologic patients is significantly less than 120 steps per minute. Walking slowly with a fluid, symmetrically alternating gait is nearly impossible at a pace less than 80 steps per minute.[216] As soon as the pace drops below 120 steps per minute, walking becomes less efficient and requires significantly more strength and balance.

The hip flexors provide a good example of how more strength is required at a pace of less than 120 steps per minute. Walking at a normal pace requires hardly any activity of the hip flexors. Walking more slowly requires the hip flexors to develop sufficient strength to actively advance the leg, which weighs about 10 kg or 22 lb. This problem is often encountered in the neurologic rehabilitation of patients with multiple sclerosis who often face difficulty in bringing their leg forward in the swing phase of the gait cycle. Findings in patients with multiple sclerosis frequently include weakness in the hip flexors as well as in the foot dorsiflexors. This means that even slight weakness in the foot dorsiflexors and hip flexors can result in a multiplier effect and lead to a major functional problem.

Other examples of weak muscles in the lower extremities in neurologic patients include the foot dorsiflexors and plantar flexors. These two muscle groups are often affected in neurologic patients. This becomes apparent when the gait immediately improves once a proper foot orthosis is used. A crucial design criterion for orthoses in neurology is that they must have a minimal weight to be effective. Therefore, it is not only important for training to increase maximum strength; in neurology, it is far more important to train muscular endurance.

The most common goal in neurologic rehabilitation, namely improving gait, can only be achieved when not only strength but also muscular endurance is well developed. Neurologic patients exhibit loss of control of the knees more frequently and prominently when they have to negotiate stairs or are tired. This is because climbing stairs requires twice as much muscle strength as walking on a leveled surface.[287] Preventing hyperextension of the knee also depends on the two factors of strength and muscular endurance.

3.3 Endurance

> **Definition** [ ]
>
> Endurance is the ability to perform a motor action as long as possible, delay the loss of performance due to fatigue, followed by a rapid recovery.

In training, various aspects of endurance may be differentiated depending on one's perspective.[88] The goal of training general endurance in recreational sports and particularly in working with neurologic patients is to ensure the development and maintenance of health.

> **Note**
>
> Endurance training is conducted at a constant level of intensity that must lie below the anaerobic threshold.

The continuous method, involving a constant level of intensity or speed, is usually employed for endurance training. The duration of exercise should be about 20 to 30 minutes. If the patient is unable to perform continuous exercise, training utilizes an interval method, consisting of high-intensity exercises for short intervals with relatively short resting periods. In the therapy of neurologic patients, exercise intensity is determined by the heart rate training zone, which is calculated using Karvonen's formula (Chapter 6.2): lower load threshold = (220 − age − pulse at rest) × 0.4 + pulse at rest; upper load threshold = (220 − age − pulse at rest) × 0.85 + pulse at rest.[263] The effect of training on endurance is primarily dependent on the duration of training and not the intensity of training. In sports, this training is used to improve basic endurance, which is also a natural goal in neurologic patients.

3.3.1 Endurance Training in Neurologic Rehabilitation

Many neurologic patients also suffer from cardiovascular problems due to their age or disability (Parkinson's disease, stroke), which in turn, often lead to endurance problems.

As was discussed earlier, a measure of endurance plays an important role in walking. A neurologic patient will not be able to walk outside the home without a certain minimal endurance in the sense of cardiovascular endurance. Patients lacking this are limited in their opportunities for social participation. Neurologic patients are often unable to walk the same distances as able-bodied people due to their physical deficits. As a result, their cardiovascular system is not trained sufficiently in daily life. This, in turn, leads to reduced endurance, resulting in a vicious circle. It is important not to confuse endurance with muscular endurance. Nor is endurance training so important in young patients with multiple sclerosis who are able to walk and actively participate in sports.

3.4 Speed

> **Definition** [ ]
>
> Speed refers to the motor ability of the brain to produce a quick motor response.

Functional musculature (strength) and neuromuscular coordination are required to allow quick execution of the movement, for example, protective steps or balance reactions.

3.4.1 Speed Training in Neurologic Rehabilitation

Speed is important for various aspects of everyday activities; it especially plays a crucial role in gait. A neurologic patient walking at 1.0 km/h (0.6 mph) needs more endurance and time to arrive at his or her destination than when walking at a normal speed. But even this patient wants to reach that destination as quickly and easily as possible. As a result, these patients switch to a wheelchair owing to a lack of sufficient strength and endurance; their environment usually provides enough time to them. The most important factor for walking outside the home after endurance is speed. Thus, it is advisable that gait training, as task-oriented training, should also aim to increase speed. This can be achieved effectively on the treadmill or by measuring times.

> **Note**
>
> Speed is also required in balance reactions to quickly execute a protective step or protective reaction. In this sense, the postural instability of patients with Parkinson's disease actually reflects a motor speed deficit.

The same rule applies to the upper extremity. Patients who can perform an action more quickly have better motor performance despite the fact that it may not appear so at the beginning of the practice situation. For this reason, exercises consisting of tasks, such as opening a bottle, eating a spoonful of peas, or unscrewing a cap, should not only be repeated often but should also be timed. This means counting the repetitions in a certain time duration (3 minutes) so that the patient is encouraged to perform them more quickly. A common drawback is that this concentrates on the quantity at the expense of quality. However, this is not the case, as findings of motor learning research have shown that quicker execution of a task can only be achieved by improving the quality of the motor function.

3.5 Mobility

> **Definition**   [ ]
>
> Mobility or flexibility comprises two components: joint mobility (range of motion) and the elasticity of the structures surrounding the joint (muscles, tendons, and capsule).

3.5.1 Promoting Elasticity and Joint Mobility in Neurologic Rehabilitation

The elasticity of the musculature is decisive when tone is increased. The literature contains conflicting information about the pathophysiology of spasticity. What is certain is that the muscle spindle reflex (gamma receptor reflex) plays an important role. The gamma receptor response means that activation or deactivation of the intrafusal muscle spindles, which measures factors, such as length and changes in the musculature, leads to increased tone or spasticity at the level of spinal cord. However, studies have also shown that a lesion of the upper motor neuron results in an intrinsic change in the muscle–tendon apparatus.[89,191,284] Adequate treatment thus includes stretching. It is advisable to perform this stretching in the sense of nerve tension. This means not just stretching the course of the muscles but also mobilization in the course of the nerve.

Example: Leg

Example for stretching the lower extremity: stretching the hamstrings including the lower leg (▶ Fig. 3.2 and ▶ Fig. 3.3).

The patient lies supine on a broad couch (either on a bed or on the floor during house calls). The therapist stands next to the leg to be stretched. The posterior thigh muscles are maximally pre-stretched by flexing the hip. With patient's foot in dorsiflexion, the therapist extends the patient's knee while maintaining the flexion in the hip. The patient determines the limit of mobilization, and the therapist must always respect this limit. When the other leg is drawn into hip flexion, the therapist can hold the leg in extension by fixing the leg with his or her foot but must immediately release the leg if this triggers sudden spasticity (▶ Fig. 3.4).

Example: Arm

Example for stretching the upper extremity: stretching with the elbow and wrist in extension; fingers may be extended as in the Elvey upper limb tension test (▶ Fig. 3.5 and ▶ Fig. 3.6).[50]

The description of the test refers to the right arm. The patient lies supine on the couch, a bit closer to

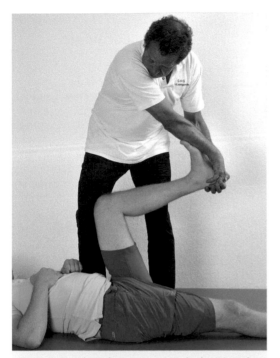

Fig. 3.2 Stretching the posterior muscle chain (initial position).

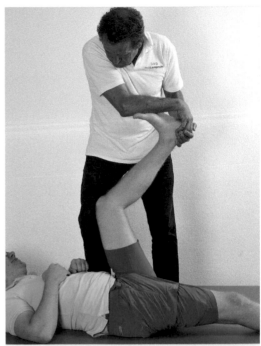

Fig. 3.3 Stretching the posterior muscle chain (final position).

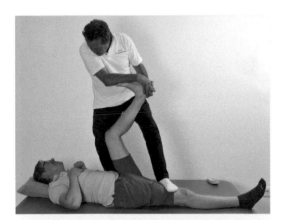

Fig. 3.4 Monitoring patient's evasive mechanisms.

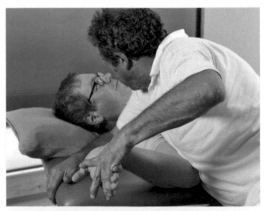

Fig. 3.5 Stretching for the upper extremity.

the right side. The patient can rest his or her head on a pillow. The therapist stands facing the patient with his or her legs apart. The therapist grasps the patient's right hand with his/her own left hand. The upper arm can be placed on the thigh. With the right hand, the therapist prevents elevation of the patient's shoulder. The patient's arm is brought into about 110 degrees of abduction. The

therapist can bring the patient's arm into abduction by taking a step if the arm rests on the therapist's thigh. The therapist now moves the patient's forearm into supination and the wrist and fingers into extension. The shoulder is now externally rotated. With the patient held in this position, mobilization can now be performed with the elbow in extension. Evasive movements by the patient

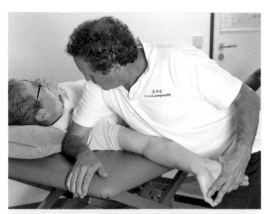

Fig. 3.6 Stretching with the elbow and wrist in extension; fingers may be extended as in the Elvey upper limb tension test.

can include extension in the cervical spine, lateral flexion to the right, or rotation to the left.[50]

3.6 Coordination

Definition	[ ]
Coordination can be described as the ability to perform different motion sequences quickly, precisely, and under different conditions.	

Why are we able to touch a finger to our nose with our eyes closed? Why are we able to walk in the dark without falling? These maneuvers require sensorimotor processes. Any movement naturally requires initial muscular activity. Reception of sensory stimuli from various receptors makes it possible to continue movements and optimize them. Due to its complexity, coordination is the basic motor skill that is most difficult to measure.

3.6.1 Coordination Training in Neurologic Rehabilitation

All neurologic patients have coordination problems to some degree. Examination findings are important in training patients with coordination problems to know the areas where coordination problems are likely to occur.

3.7 Balance

Definition	[ ]
Balance can be described as the state in which the forces acting on the body cancel each other out.[215] Balance can be either static or dynamic.	

3.7.1 Balance Training in Neurologic Rehabilitation

There is no uniform nomenclature for describing exercises to improve postural control. Some authors refer to "balance training."[27,168,396] Others use the terms "sensorimotor training,"[17,153] "neuromuscular training,"[295] or "proprioceptive training."

Balance is a key topic in neurologic rehabilitation, as neurologic disorders frequently lead to impaired balance. The impairment of balance can have a variety of causes depending on the affected structures and the underlying disorders. The effects of impaired balance invariably include increased risk of falling and reduced mobility.[21,208] For a person to maintain his/her balance, there must be a system that is able to detect the forces acting on the body as well as activate muscles and initiate movement programs to compensate for these incident forces. The sensorimotor system is just such a system.[337,338] Examination findings are crucial to the success of balance training, as they help to find out the structures primarily responsible for the balance impairment. The ability to maintain balance is related to activity and is trainable at any age.[150]

In therapeutic exercise, all these basic motor skills are trained in precisely the manner that optimizes the benefit patients receive.

Under normal physiological conditions, the basic motor skills are closely intertwined. All the skills should be optimally developed and trained to achieve an optimal result.

The neurologic deficit influences the result of training. Even training therapy is unable to reverse the fact of the disorder or injury. Neurologic patients can only achieve training results within the scope dictated by their disorder and its severity. Nonetheless, an adequately designed training program can train all basic motor skills and improve the motor outcome.

4 Neurologic Rehabilitation

"A genius! For 37 years I have practiced 14 hours a day, and now they are calling me a genius!"
(P. Sarasate, Spanish violinist, 1848–1908)

4.1 Cortical Reorganization

The rehabilitation of neurologic patients aims to restore the greatest possible independence within the limits dictated by the disability. Spontaneous, at least partial improvement of the motor, cognitive, and/or perceptive deficits, is often observed following damage to the central nervous system (CNS). This means that the CNS must be able to compensate for this damage in some way.

Increasing number of studies have greatly improved our understanding of neuronal reorganization, and neurologic rehabilitation has changed dramatically in response to these new findings. The ability of the CNS to reorganize its neuronal structure enables it to relearn capabilities and compensate for brain injuries by means of reorganizing cortical and subcortical networks. Studies suggest that functional reorganization of the motor cortex occurs both as a result of a lesion in the central or peripheral nervous system (lesion-induced plasticity) and as a consequence of motor training (training-induced plasticity).[111,384] Training-induced plasticity can also be understood as use-related plasticity. Following a brain injury, both lesion-induced plasticity and use-induced plasticity are operative and mesh with each other. The simple repetition of the same movement is not only a requirement for motor learning, it is also a requirement for cortical reorganization in the sense of "practice makes perfect" or "use it or lose it."[235]

Plasticity may be regarded as the ability of the CNS to adapt structurally and functionally to altered demands.[45] This means that the old notions of a hierarchically structured CNS and of a peripheral nervous system that acts as the uppermost control organ are no longer tenable. We now know that the central and peripheral nervous systems constantly interact with each other and adapt via feedback systems to the respective new situations. "Form changes in response to a change in function. Function changes in response to a change in form."[205]

With the introduction of the International Classification of Functioning, Disability, and Health (ICF) by the World Health Organization (WHO) in 2001, the goals of neurologic rehabilitation have changed. The ICF replaced the earlier International Classification of Impairment, Disability, and Handicap (ICIDH). A purely biomedical model has thus been replaced by a biopsychosocial model (2005), thereby shifting the focus in neurologic rehabilitation to participation in social life (▶ Fig. 4.1).[137] In the last few years, this has brought about a paradigm shift in the rehabilitation of persons with neurologic symptoms.

> **Note**
>
> The "classic" therapy methods, such as those of Bobath, Vojta, proprioceptive neuromuscular facilitation, etc. are paving the way for newer evidence-based therapy concepts; what was once a confession is now becoming a profession.[187]

Scientific research has shown that these new methods and therapy concepts have successfully produced certain effects in neurologic patients. Both basic experimental research and randomized studies are crucial to the development and evaluation of rehabilitation concepts and methods.[89] These demonstrations of efficacy are subjected to the clear rules of the natural sciences. A hierarchy of evidence applies, which is clearly determined by the degree of evidence (▶ Fig. 4.2).

However, this does not mean that the "old" therapy methods should no longer be used simply because there are too few studies or no convincing studies that demonstrate the efficacy of these "traditional" methods. Yet, these treatment techniques and concepts will only retain their validity in neurologic rehabilitation if they are able to integrate the new findings about motor learning. Nonetheless, it should be noted that it is very difficult to scientifically validate the therapeutic methods in physical therapy, as therapy studies are easily contested.

Heidi Höppner, the first woman professor at the Department of Physical Therapy at the University of Kiel, noted at a Physioaustria Congress: "Whether purely scientific criteria are in keeping with the essence of physical therapy is open to question." This statement seeks to

The ICF biopsychosocial model

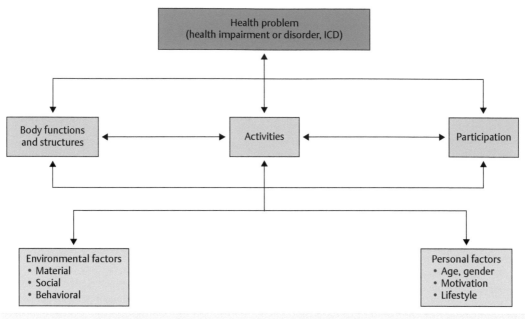

Fig. 4.1 International Classification of Functioning, Disability, and Health (ICF), 2005.

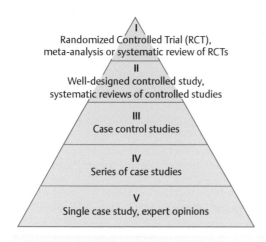

Fig. 4.2 Hierarchy of evidence.

express how difficult it is to perform a physiotherapeutic therapy study whose methodology cannot be questioned.

It is very difficult to obtain evidence in an open concept such as the Bobath concept, as the therapist's personality is one of the decisive factors influencing the patient's reaction. Evidence-based studies fail to take the importance of these interactions between therapist and patient into consideration. Nonetheless, the rehabilitation of patients with CNS disorders will have to conform to the principles of motor learning processes in the future. It will not be enough to simply apply the terminology of motor learning to existing concepts while continuing to follow the same principles as 30 years ago.

Learning is a process of acquiring new experiences and skills. There are two basic forms of learning: explicit and implicit learning. Learning motor skills primarily involves the implicit components; the explicit components are merely secondary. Relearning movements is understood as a hands-on learning process that neurologic patients must master by themselves with minimal assistance from their therapists. The therapist's primary task in neurologic rehabilitation is to guide the patients to various forms of training to provide them ample opportunity for independent training (▶ Fig. 4.3). Recent studies have demonstrated that the patient's ability to influence the sequence of exercises has a positive effect on the acquisition of motor skills.[443]

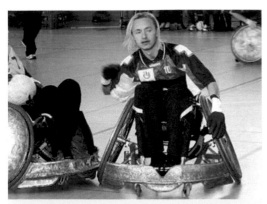

Fig. 4.3 Activity for neurologic patients: wheelchair rugby.

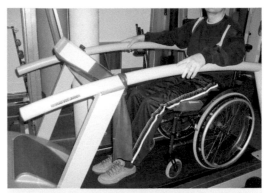

Fig. 4.4 A patient mobilized in a wheelchair should learn to walk again.

Note

There is also evidence to suggest that individual therapy is not necessarily always optimal and that therapy in pairs or even in larger groups can be more effective. This is attributed to the fact that patients who practice in groups benefit from observing other patients and are able to copy motor strategies more comfortably from them.

A social effect is also observable in such groups; patients are more strongly motivated and compete among themselves. The cost–benefit ratio is also better in pairs or groups than in the individual therapy. These effects have only been demonstrated for neurologic patients in a few studies, although the data for other groups of patients are very reliable.[443]

4.1.1 Primary Goals in Motor Rehabilitation

In the ICF framework, the primary goals are to promote independence and personal mobility; maintain and improve social integration (family, social setting, work); improve quality of life; improve and/or eliminate symptoms and disabilities; and reduce the intensity of care in neurologic rehabilitation.

On the whole, this involves a shift from passive or guided therapy situations toward therapy forms involving active exercises. Recent studies on motor rehabilitation demonstrate that those therapeutic approaches and techniques whose concepts involve high-intensity training and active, task-oriented motion training are superior to traditional methods of treatment. This means that the patient in bed is mobilized out of bed, the patient mobilized in a wheelchair learns to walk again (▶ Fig. 4.4), and the walking patient learns to walk with greater speed and confidence, even under the conditions of daily life. What is crucial is not that patients master a task but that they repeat the task frequently and independently.

While planning the therapy, it is crucial to pay attention to the transfer from therapy to the patient's daily life. It is clear that this transfer does not take place automatically meaning that the therapist must become aware of this transfer issue so that he or she can critically examine the content of the therapy.[247] When examining one's own therapy content, the therapist should follow the Skaggs–Robinson curve and keep in mind that motor learning is invariably specific. Consequently, the training itself must be specific and task related (▶ Fig. 4.5).[190] Huber explains the importance of training in everyday situations. He also demonstrates that the decisive factors in a successful transfer include the similarity of motor sequences and the underlying neuronal processes.

The Skaggs–Robinson curve illustrates the recognized theory that no interplay exists between the two completely different task classes. Transfer is most effective when the exercise sequence is identical to the target movement. If the situation lies between these two extremes and the exercise bears slight similarity to the target movement, then, strangely, negative interplay can occur. The patient's motor system is unable to react and attempts

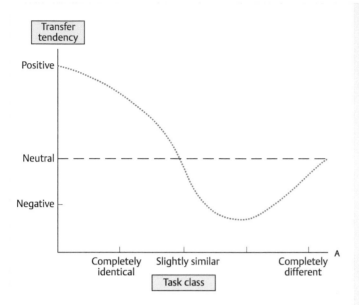

Fig. 4.5 Transfer problem: Therapy bench-walking.

to apply inexpedient motion components to the new task situation. Huber illustrates these transfer situations with the example of children learning to ride a bicycle. Children who have previously practiced with a kick scooter usually master bicycle riding more quickly and easily than children who begin to ride with training wheels. This is because on the scooter, children are precisely able to achieve the balance that they need on a bicycle. Training wheels, on the other hand, prevent rather than promote many typical movements in bicycle riding. For example, it is not possible to lean into a curve when the inside training wheel prevents it.[190]

Putting this into practice means that treatment should focus on everyday situations, as the motor learning processes are identical in able-bodied persons and those with neurologic deficits.[246] This implies that the same models used for learning movements in sports can be successfully applied to neurologic rehabilitation.

Note

Essential factors for the success of motor learning include:
- Motivation of the person involved.
- Number of repetitions.
- Applicability to daily life situations.
- A therapy situation conducive to learning.
- Continually increasing the requirement.
- Frequency and type of feedback about the respective success.

These general principles of motor learning originated from sports and training research and have been scientifically proven for many years. These fundamental principles of functional, goal-oriented exercise were introduced into neurologic rehabilitation by Carr and Shepherd as a "motor relearning program" in 1987.

4.1.2 Modern Approaches and Concepts in Neurologic Rehabilitation

Constraint-Induced Movement Therapy

Constraint-induced movement therapy (CIMT)[395,439] may be mentioned first. "Forced use" is a therapy concept primarily used in treating arm deficits in patients with hemiparesis. The therapy attempts to reverse the "learned nonuse" of the hand or arm or even prevent it from occurring. The origin of this was the forced use therapy whose effectiveness Ostendorf and Wolf[129] had demonstrated in 1981. This involved immobilizing the unaffected extremity for several hours over a period of 2 weeks. In addition to the immobilization, Taub et al[394] and Miltner et al[269] conducted repetitive training of functionally relevant arm movements in the affected extremity. The authors referred to this procedure as "constraint-induced movement therapy (CIMT)."[129] In this method, the patient is "forced" to use the hemiparetic hand or arm in everyday activities. This is achieved by neutralizing or impeding the use of the normal hand by means of a forearm splint or a glove.

The concept proceeds from the premise that in patients with hemiplegia, a quicker, more sustainable improvement in the function of the affected arm can be achieved by intensive stimulation of the repair processes in the brain (neuroplasticity). The forced use of the affected arm prevents the learned nonuse of it. The principles of CIMT are consistent with the modern theories of motor learning. The effective components of CIMT include intensive repetitive exercise, task-oriented exercise in everyday situations, and continuous adaptation of the requirement to the patient's current level of performance (shaping).

With their working group, Wolf and Taub demonstrated the efficacy of this therapeutic approach in the rehabilitation of arm and hand function in patients who had suffered a stroke.[440] After a 2-week-period of 6 hours of treatment per day, the improvement persisted even 24 months after the therapy. However, this study was conducted with a highly selective group of patients who were required to fulfill very specific and strict requirements. It is not known how many patients with chronic stroke actually fulfill these requirements. For this reason, studies have been performed in recent years to determine the extent to which CIMT could be modified to adapt it to the concept of clinical rehabilitation practice in Germany.[89]

Dettmers et al[84] reduced the intensity of the repetitive exercise to 3 hours per day while increasing the duration of rehabilitation to 4 weeks or more. Good rehabilitation results have also been achieved with this strategy. Dromerick[98] has shown the positive effect of CIMT in acute and subacute poststroke phases. Gordon et al[148] demonstrated that children with cerebral palsy and a primarily unilateral motor deficit can also benefit from CIMT (▶Fig. 4.6).

CIMT has proved beneficial, especially in the upper extremity where function in one hand or arm is impaired, and patients tend to completely avoid using the affected extremity, such that the patient effectively has only one working hand. Comparing the function of the upper and lower extremities, we often find the lower extremity to perform everyday functions in a significantly better way than the upper extremity. This means that although a patient with hemiparesis is often capable of walking, the affected arm remains nonfunctional, as the patient effectively has one working hand. One reason for this is "learned nonuse." If the person attempts to use the hand or arm, it may lead to

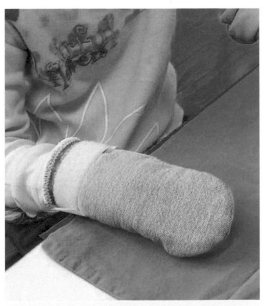

Fig. 4.6 Child with a custom glove to restrict the use of the hand.

failure and frustration. The CNS interprets this as a strategy that does not produce results whenever the healthy side is used; it invariably leads to the desired result. This results in a more prominent representation of the unaffected hand or arm and to a reduced representation of the affected hand or arm (▶ Fig. 4.7). In the lower extremity, this is simply impossible due to the alternating use of both legs when walking.

Hamzei et al modified CIMT for the lower extremity. In contrast to the CIMT concept of immobilizing the less affected hand, the less affected leg was not immobilized. Instead, the principle of "shaping" was applied to intensive gait training, for which the authors introduced the term "shaping-induced movement therapy (SIMT)."[161] The intervention was conducted over 2 consecutive weeks for 6 hours each day. All patients, and primarily chronic stroke patients, improved significantly in all the measured parameters. Thus, Hamzei et al demonstrated that intensive therapy could bring about a significant improvement in mobility even years after a stroke. The crucial factor is the intensity of training.

In neurologic patients, the effect of learned nonuse is observed not only in arm and hand function but also in leg and foot function. Other examples of learned nonuse include trunk activity in patients on wheelchair. Therefore, our most intensive everyday trunk training is walking. Walking 10,000 steps a day means 10,000 three-dimensional exercises for all of the musculature of the trunk in a functional context. A few exercises in the therapy session cannot be a substitute for this intensive training. Therefore, patients using a wheelchair should walk as often as possible, for example, on the treadmill in therapy, and otherwise stand as often as possible, if necessary in a standing frame, preferably a mobile one. A neurologic patient who is unable to walk on his own should stand for at least 1 hour each day (▶ Fig. 4.8).

Another example of learned nonuse is walking. A patient facing great difficulty in walking or for whom walking is very slow and strenuous will often walk less and repeatedly use a wheelchair to get to his/her destinations. Walking tend to worsen significantly as the patient practices considerably less. The entire musculature required for walking is no longer trained as a group, and a few exercises of individual muscle groups have little to no effect. A neurologic patient who does not walk outside the home must be encouraged to walk at home as much as possible; the patient may even purchase a treadmill.

Walking worsens as a result of learned nonuse. Three years after a stroke, 21% of stroke patients were found to have reduced mobility (a decrease of 2 or more points according to the Rivermead Mobility Index).[412] compared with the findings at the end of rehabilitation. This high number is presumably attributable to the fact that patients walk too little in their home environment. The fact that rehabilitation fails to prepare patients sufficiently for their personal environment contributes to the high number. The principles of motor learning apply here too, and according to the law of identical

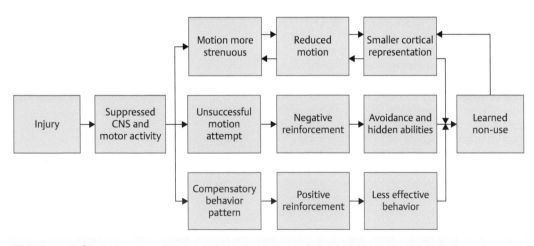

Fig. 4.7 Learned non-use.

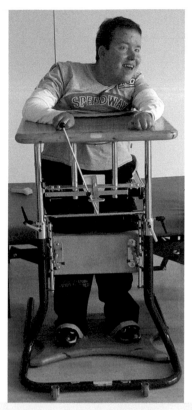

Fig. 4.8 Standing using a standing device.

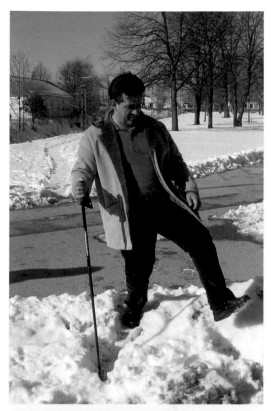

Fig. 4.9 Stroke patient: walking in snow.

elements, patients must practice walking outside the home under precisely the same conditions as they encounter at home, i.e., uphill and downhill, dual task, or on different surfaces (▶Fig. 4.9).[246]

Repetitive Sensorimotor Hand Training

Repetitive sensorimotor hand training is another new concept. In the repetitive sensorimotor hand training presented by Bütefisch et al in 1995, the patient performs simple, regularly repetitive motions of hands and fingers for the upper extremity affected by CNS paresis. These are repeated as often as possible in two daily 15-minute sessions over a period of 1 to 4 weeks. The strength and speed requirements are continuously adapted to the patient's increasing level of performance (shaping). The patient initially performs movements that he or she has already mastered, such as making a fist or dorsiflexing the wrist. A series of new movements are later introduced into the training

program. Patients demonstrated decreased spasticity and increased mobility after training.[49]

Impairment-Oriented Training

Impairment-oriented training (IOT) provides for two methods of therapy:
- Arm ability training for patients with slight paresis.
- Arm basis training for patients with severe paresis.

Platz et al[315] developed this concept for the rehabilitation of poststroke arm paresis based on three elements: First, the impairments responsible for the limitation of arm activity are clinically and neurologically analyzed. Next, specific training is developed based on these data. Finally, the efficacy of these training interventions is verified.[309] As patients exhibit either slight paralysis or severe paresis in the arm after a stroke, Platz et al[315] have described two different forms of IOT:
- Arm basis training
- Arm ability training

Patients with slight arm paresis exhibit a nearly normal active range of motion. They have nearly normal strength and can use their arm in many daily activities. However, it was demonstrated that these patients are impaired in their motor control with respect to speed and precision in various motor tasks requiring diverse sensorimotor abilities.[314] These patients are slower and less coordinated and therefore need more time and energy for performing daily activities that require the use of the arm.[308]

The arm ability training addresses precisely these difficulties. Both speed and precision are trained. The structured and repetitive design of the training promotes motor learning; introduction of variations in the exercises helps one to know whether the improved function transfers well into daily life. The tasks in the arm ability training program are selected to stimulate the various sensorimotor abilities. Therefore, training should invariably include the entire program. The important thing is that the exercises are performed with good precision as quickly as possible. The evaluation places greater emphasis on the motor performance than the manner of execution.

Arm basis training was developed by C. Eickhoff for patients with severe arm paresis.[108] Patients with severe arm paresis can hardly use their arm in everyday situations or at the best have very limited use of it. These patients suffer from the problem of unable to stabilize or move individual segments. The main problem these patients face is the lack of strength and coordination in various ranges of the desired movement.[2] Arm basis training is divided into three steps:

- First, selective innervation for isolated movements without holding activity.
- Next, selective innervation for isolated movements with holding activity.
- Only then, selective innervation for complex movements with holding activity.

In each step, the various degrees of freedom of the arm are repetitively exercised.

Strength Training

Until recently, it was unthinkable to advocate strength training in neurology, let alone offer it to patients (Chapter 3). The last few years have witnessed a sharp increase in the number of publications about strength training in connection with various neurologic clinical pictures (▶Fig. 4.10).[366,425,434,449,72,349,119]

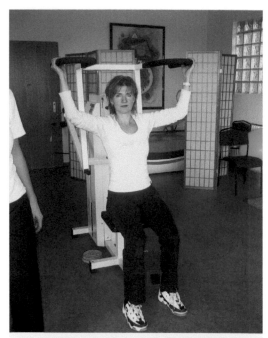

Fig. 4.10 Strength training for neurologic patients.

Naturally, strength training must be adapted to the clinical picture and the severity of the disability. Nonetheless, it is important to train all aspects of strength even with neurologic patients, naturally with the focus on muscular endurance (Chapter 3 and Chapter 7).

Bilateral Training

Bilateral training is another validated concept whose goal is to facilitate function in the paretic extremity by mirror image activity of the unaffected contralateral side.[428] This concept was primarily developed for the upper extremities. Bilateral training involves performing many repetitions bilaterally on exercise equipment. Equipment for bilateral arm training include devices such as the Bi-Manu-Track, Reha-Slide, and Reha-Slide Duo (▶Fig. 4.13). These three devices were combined with the Reha-Digit from Hesse and Buschfort to form the concept of the arm laboratory.[48]

The Bi-Manu-Track is based on a distal approach. With the distal approach in poststroke rehabilitation of the upper extremity, there is evidence to suggest that a proximal inhibition leads to a significant improvement in hand function in stroke patients. The larger cortical representation of the hand and fingers also favors a distal approach in the rehabilitation of the upper extremity. The Bi-Manu-Track trains pronation and supination of the forearm and wrist flexion and dorsiflexion bilaterally; the patient can train both movements actively and passively.

The design of the Bi-Manu-Track ensures smooth motion. Resistance, speed, and amplitude can be adjusted separately for each side so that training with the Bi-Manu-Track can be adapted individually to the patient's performance (▶Fig. 4.11).[177] The Reha-Slide is a mechanical device for training

elbow flexion and extension; shoulder abduction and adduction; and wrist flexion and dorsiflexion. Software presets are available for many therapeutic tasks (▶Fig. 4.12).

The Reha-Slide-Duo is a purely mechanical device for patients who already have a certain degree of function in the hand and arm. The resistance can be adjusted separately for each side, and the hand grips can also be adjusted separately to adapt to the functional problems (▶Fig. 4.13).

The Reha-Digit was developed to stimulate finger movement. The patient places his or her fingers (without the thumb) into a device with a moving shaft, which passively moves the fingers. The combined effect of stimulating the fingertips together with the vibratory stimulus integrated into the unit provides a maximum of sensory stimulation (▶Fig. 4.14).

Robot-Assisted Training

One of the new concepts of neurologic rehabilitation is the robot-assisted training. Therapy robots have been developed for training both the upper and lower extremities. As early as 1995, Hogan et al[182] introduced the MIT Manus, a robot that can perform passive movements in the elbow and shoulder in the horizontal plane. The Mirror Image Movement Enabler (MIME) robot utilizes the bilateral approach to train movements in the elbow and shoulder of the affected side. The healthy side defines the movement, and the affected side follows.[240]

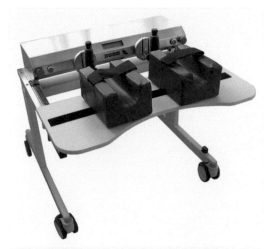

Fig. 4.11 Bi-Manu-Track. Used with the kind permission of Reha-Stim Medtec GmbH & Co. KG, Berlin, Germany.

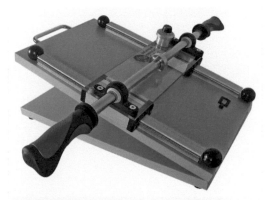

Fig. 4.12 Reha-Slide. Used with the kind permission of Reha-Stim Medtec GmbH & Co. KG, Berlin, Germany.

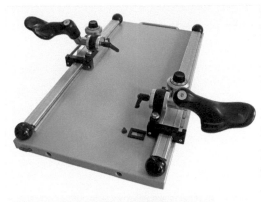

Fig. 4.13 Reha-Slide Duo. Used with the kind permission of Reha-Stim Medtec GmbH & Co. KG, Berlin, Germany.

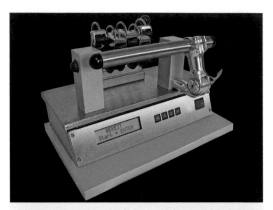

Fig. 4.14 Reha-Digit for finger mobilization. Used with the kind permission of Reha-Stim Medtec GmbH & Co. KG, Berlin, Germany.

Modern robots for training the upper extremities have far more degrees of freedom, thereby allowing very realistic training in conjunction with virtual reality. Examples of these robots include the Amadeo Rehabilitation (▶Fig. 4.15), Armeo Spring, and Armeo Power (▶Fig. 4.16). The common thing in these rehabilitation robots is the capacity for conducting highly repetitive training with the patient. The training is precisely adapted according to various degrees of difficulty and based on automatically collected data. These data are also used to document the progress of the patient.

With the appropriate software, the Pablo system allows precisely defined movements and grasping training of the arm and hand (▶Fig. 4.17). New developments in training arm, hand, and finger function have entered the market. The units have become progressively smaller while the range of uses has become ever larger and more specific. An example of this is the YouGrabber from YouRehab. A particular advantage of the YouGrabber is the option of unilateral or bilateral training. Certain problem areas can be selectively trained, or training can include hand–arm coordination or both arms (▶Fig. 4.18). The last few years have witnessed rapid strides in the development of new computerized therapy options for treating sensorimotor deficits in the upper extremities. The common aspect of these therapy options is that they employ game elements and a computer connection to significantly extend the training time.

Currently, many robots are available in the market for training the lower extremities. Two approaches can be observed with gait trainers, namely, foot-controlled and leg-controlled gait trainers. The foot-controlled gait trainers include the electromagnetic gait trainer, GT I. The patient is secured with a belt and stands on two footplates whose movement simulates the stance and swing phases. This movement also stimulates the vertical and lateral shifts in the body's center of gravity in the respective phases of the gait cycle that are needed for walking (▶Fig. 4.19). The LokoHelp is another foot-controlled gait trainer. Both feet of the patient are fitted with orthoses that are then attached to the LokoHelp. There is an option for body-weight support where indicated. Patients can also practice walking uphill with the

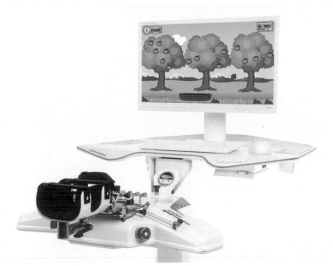

Fig. 4.15 Amadeo-Rehabilitation for the finger and hand. Used with the kind permission of Tyromotion GmbH, Graz, Austria.

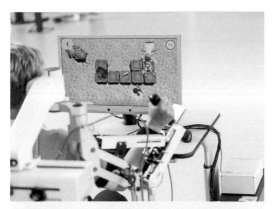

Fig. 4.16 Armeo spring allows three-dimensional movement in virtual reality as well. Used with the kind permission of Hocoma, Volketswil, Switzerland.

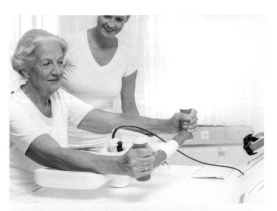

Fig. 4.17 Patient training with the Pablo system. Used with the kind permission of Tyromotion GmbH, Graz, Austria.

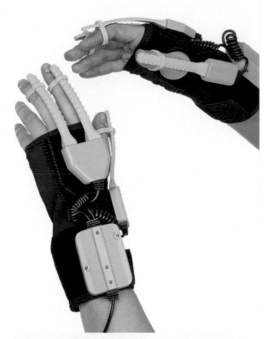

Fig. 4.18 YouGrabber training. Used with the kind permission of YouRehab AG, Schlieren, Switzerland.

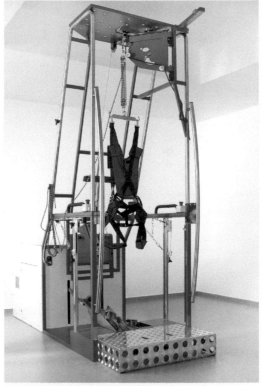

Fig. 4.19 Treadmill training with the GT I. Used with the kind permission of Reha-Stim Medtec GmbH & Co. KG, Berlin, Germany.

LokoHelp (▶Fig. 4.20). The Robowalk expander supplied by h/p/cosmos provides a simple design for assisted walking (▶Fig. 4.21).

The leg-controlled gait trainers include the Lokomat. The system consists of a powered gait orthosis that automates guidance of the legs of gait-impaired patients on the treadmill (▶Fig. 4.22).

The Heidelberg University Medical Center is pursuing a completely new development, where researchers are working on MoreGait, a walking robot for the home. The patient can undergo gait training in a semireclining position (BMBF).[34] The MoreGait utilizes pneumatic muscles to provide patients only as much assistance as they need. Patients must exhaust their own capabilities before receiving assistance from the robot (▶ Fig. 4.23).

The Erigo is a tilting table with an integral leg drive unit; this allows severely affected patients who still lack stable cardiovascular function to repetitively train intensive functional leg movements in an increasingly vertical position (▶ Fig. 4.24).

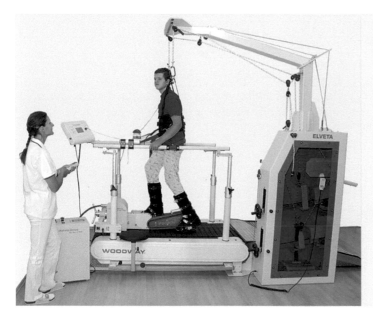

Fig. 4.20 LokoHelp. Used with the kind permission of www.lokohelp.net.

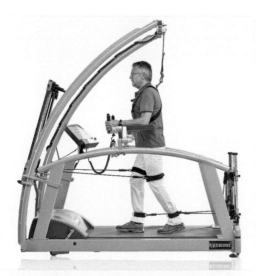

Fig. 4.21 Robowalk expander. Used with the kind permission of h/p/cosmos sports & medical GmbH, Nussdorf-Traunstein, Germany.

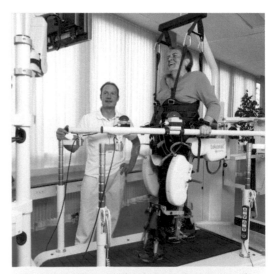

Fig. 4.22 Lokomat. Used with the kind permission of Hocoma, Switzerland.

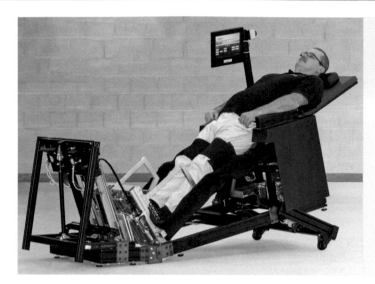

Fig. 4.23 MoreGait. Used with the kind permission of Clinic for Paraplegiology of the Heidelberg University Medical Center, Heidelberg, Germany.

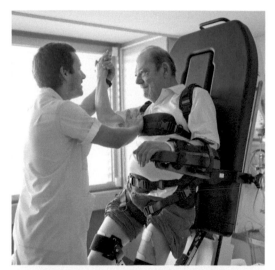

Fig. 4.24 Erigo, tilting table for early rehabilitation. Used with the kind permission of Hocoma, Volketswil, Switzerland.

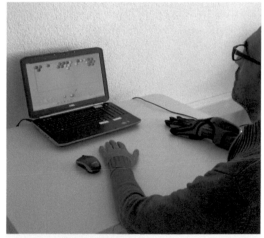

Fig. 4.25 Virtual reality.

Patients who can already walk but are still at a risk of falling can benefit from partial weight-bearing systems, as the repetition of the gait cycle is significantly higher than when walking on a leveled surface.

Virtual Reality Training

Virtual reality training is another evidence-based treatment concept. Patients with a distally pronounced paresis demonstrated improvement in all aspects of trained movements following a 2-week period of virtual reality training. The patients wore special glove that measured all finger movements (▶ Fig. 4.25). The movements measured were then transferred to a realistic image of a hand on the monitor. The task consisted of mastering certain repetitive movements. The demands were adapted to the patient's current level of performance.[266]

Mirror Therapy

Altschuler et al[9] published an article in 1999 in which they described a positive effect of mirror therapy in poststroke patients. Since then, many studies have demonstrated the benefit of mirror therapy in the rehabilitation of arm paresis following stroke (▶ Fig. 4.26).[401]

For many years, imagining the motion has been an integral part of the overall training plan for learning motor sequences in sports and in occupational settings, for example, among musicians, pilots, and ballet dancers. Mental practice has only been tried in the neurologic rehabilitation of CNS lesions for a few years.[256] Imagined movements activate the same areas in the CNS as an actual active movement.[291] Observing the movement also activates the same areas as performing the movement. The more familiar the observed movement is, the stronger is the activity in the mirror neurons of the individuals observing the movement. For example, ballet dancers exhibit the highest activity in their mirror neurons when they watch other ballet dancers; yet, they exhibit a lesser degree of activity when they observe other dance performances. The conclusion for neurologic rehabilitation would be that patients should especially observe the movements they are familiar with, for example, walking and grasping. This is presumably one reason why rehabilitation can be more successful in a small group than in individual therapy.

4.2 Feedback Training

Feedback plays an important role in neurologic rehabilitation; it is important that positive feedback be provided quickly.

Feedback can be given in several ways:

- **Verbal feedback:** It is important to avoid sentences beginning with "but" in verbal feedback. One should refrain from making well-intentioned suggestions for improvement. Instead, the therapist should clearly emphasize the goal and effect of the motion and encourage the patient like an athlete.
- **Acoustic feedback:** Acoustic feedback has long been used in the neurologic rehabilitation of patients with Parkinson's disease. This acoustic feedback is now integrated into various computer-controlled training games and includes positive feedback at the end of a task.
- **Vestibular feedback:** Patients receive vestibular feedback from receptors in the inner ear whenever they change the position of their body. This can be performed easily using a training device known as SpaceCurl. The patient stands in the unit with his feet immobilized. Enabling the individual rings allows different planes of motion. When the patient shifts his weight, it immediately changes the position of his body in space, producing vestibular feedback (▶ Fig. 4.27 and ▶ Fig. 4.28).
- **Visual feedback:** Visual feedback is increasingly gaining importance. Today, visual feedback in neurologic rehabilitation is provided by computer-controlled training devices, such as Armeo, PABLO, and SilverFit (▶ Fig. 4.29) or cycling trainers.

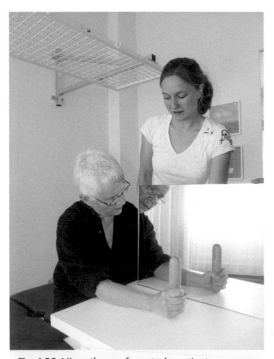

Fig. 4.26 Mirror therapy for a stroke patient.

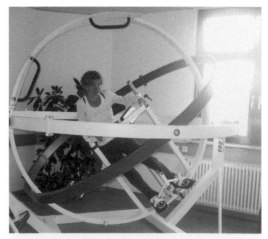

Fig. 4.27 SpaceCurl starting position.

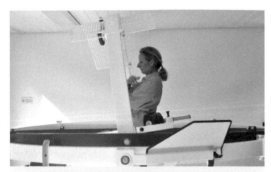

Fig. 4.28 SpaceCurl end position.

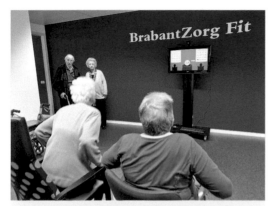

Fig. 4.29 SilverFit (Copyright 2011 SilverFit B.V./ Robert van den Berge).

Many neurologic therapy devices can be connected to a desktop PC or laptop. This provides patients with an immediate feedback as to whether their movement was performed effectively. The presets should be selected by physical therapists or sports researchers and applied with consideration given to the patient's individual problems.

When one examines the modern concepts in neurorehabilitation, it is readily apparent that one of the most important points is that each of these forms of therapy should be applied intensively with a great amount of repetition. In today's health care environment of limited financial resources, this intensity can be achieved in neither inpatient nor outpatient treatment in the one-to-one therapist–patient constellation. This implies that new ways must be found to allow as many neurologic rehabilitation patients as possible to benefit from these findings. The use of training programs adapted to the individual patient represents one such possibility.

Summary ✔

When this knowledge is applied to the therapy of patients with neurologic lesions, it becomes clear that the rehabilitation of neurologic patients must follow certain principles:
- Relevance to daily life
- Repetition
- Daily exercise at the tolerance limit
- Environment conducive to learning
- Feedback training

5 Therapeutic Exercise in Neurology: Why?

"The eye sees only what the mind already knows."
(Johann Wolfgang von Goethe)

5.1 Introduction

> **Definition** [ ]
>
> "Therapeutic exercise is the application of physical training with (still) healthy persons or patients within the scope of a preventative or curative medical treatment, as recommended and prescribed by a physician, with clear indications, in order to achieve defined therapeutic goals. Therapeutic exercise is thus the continuation of medical treatment by other means."[158]

For nearly 20 years, there have been many indications that the number of repetitions and the intensity of rehabilitation play an essential role in relearning motor skills. Raes[327] showed in her dissertation that the speed of fine motor movements is more important for motor learning than the precision of the movement. Persons who underwent fast training demonstrated more pronounced learning success in follow-up than the control group. Therapeutic exercise, in particular, provides us the opportunity to specifically and reproducibly increase the intensity and speed. Other contributing factors are that the therapy is task oriented, the patient receives proper feedback, and the training takes place at the patient's tolerance limit. This indicates that the exercises must always be adapted to the patient's level of performance (shaping).[439,192] Therapeutic exercise is able to achieve this shaping very effectively and with fine precision. Whether training on equipment is task oriented is debatable. Nonetheless, various equipment can be considered to involve a task, for example, a climbing wall. Yet, this could even apply to an elliptical trainer, exercise bicycle, and treadmill.

As was discussed in Chapter 4, a new understanding based on the points mentioned above has evolved in neurologic rehabilitation over the last few years. Therapeutic exercise includes many of the important points of the new approaches to therapy in neurologic rehabilitation. As a result, it is well suited as an important form of therapy for neurologic patients. Another advantage of therapeutic exercise can be seen from the fact that the training is not primarily associated with disease and therapy but can be viewed as "I am getting back into shape." Additional positive factor includes the social contacts that can arise in a training situation. The patients come into contact with other people, learn from observing, make new social contacts, understand that they are not alone with their problems, and can compare themselves with other affected persons. This can also lead to a certain competition. A basic element of human nature is that competition stimulates a person's own performance, especially when the differences in performance do not appear to be insurmountable. Performing better than one's neighbor increases a person's motivation to achieve new goals.

It has been shown that in Parkinson's disease, strenuous forced training improves motor function better than a training of intensity of the patient's own choice. When training intensity was set 30% higher than the intensity patients would have selected themselves, they achieved an improvement of 35% on the Unified Parkinson's Disease Rating Scale (UPDRS). Patients who trained at an intensity of their own choice improved only in the area of aerobic fitness.[336]

Motor learning occurs most effectively in the context of purposeful, targeted sequences of actions or in a functional context. This means that people learn grasping by grasping, sitting up by sitting up, standing by standing, and walking by walking. For neurologic rehabilitation, this means that implicit learning is crucial to relearning or improving a motor skill.

5.2 Factors Promoting Motor Learning

Kwakkel et al[220] demonstrated that more intensive training (massed practice) achieves a better result than less intensive training. Liepert[236] reported that the intensity and frequency of training are important for its overall success. A stimulating learning environment in which patients can recognize a relationship to their daily routine is a necessity in neurologic rehabilitation.[30] Task-specific exercises produce better results than the training that only involves individual muscles and has no connection to patients' daily life.[311,447,54]

In therapeutic exercise, this can be achieved by training involving familiar patterns, such as walking, climbing, and bicycling.

Repetitive exercise, many repetitions of individual movements, leads to an improvement in execution.[49] This means that a high number of repetitions is necessary to improve the quality of movement. With respect to walking, this also means that treadmill training will improve endurance and walking speed if the training intensity is kept sufficiently high.[173,172,427] Walking speed and endurance, in particular, are important parameters for walking outside the home. Neurologic patients only walk outside the home if they can walk long and fast enough. These quantitative improvements are coupled with qualitative improvements.

Training can be organized as circuit training meaning that exercises should alternate between strength and endurance and between the upper and lower extremities.[54] Success in neurorehabilitation also depends on an environment conducive to learning.[345,347] In neurologic rehabilitation as well as in therapeutic exercise, patients must always go as far as their tolerance limit. Performance must always be adapted in therapy and during training.[122]

Randomized practice trains adaptability to different tasks, thereby facilitating the transfer to activities of daily life and improving patient's reactions.[443] Practicing in unpredictable situations promotes and facilitates the development of effective strategies. The neurologic patient needs success in rehabilitation because successfully executed movements cause strategies to be stored in the central nervous system (CNS).[369] Success in executing movements increases motivation, which is also a requirement for mastering new tasks in the future. The therapist's instructions should not be directed toward performing the movement but the goal or effect of the movement; the task should have an external focus. This would, in turn, lead to improved efficiency of movement, decreased frequency of errors, and greater maximum strength that the patient can generate.[448,444,445,117,264] All these effects contribute to the movement becoming automatic.

Note

Well-planned pauses should be a matter of course. When simple motions are performed, the rule of thumb is that the pause should be about half as long as the time required for the exercise. For complex motions, the pause should be about twice as long as the time required for the motion.

This does not necessarily mean that there should be no activity during the pauses; the pauses can be used to train other muscle groups. Pauses in therapeutic exercise can also be put to good use for group therapy and pair training or for learning from observation and mental practice. The longest pause, sleep, is also necessary for effective motor learning.[424] Pauses are thus important but there should not be too many. One obvious reason is the limited therapy time.

Positively formulated feedback is also important for motor learning, especially when the patients themselves can choose when and how feedback is given. Wulf[443] demonstrated that the motor outcome is measurably improved by positive feedback. Feedback is given about the result, not about the execution (knowledge of results).[446,54,369]

"Motor learning is the sum of the processes, which by practice or experience, leads to relatively stable neuronal changes and consequently to skillful actions even under changing contextual conditions."[368] Schindl et al[355] demonstrated that repetition of simple motor movements was able to improve the quality and speed of a task.

As in sports, the dosage of strength and endurance training should be increased according to the principles of training research. Variability, interest, and motivation can be maintained by changing the intensity, frequency, scope, and duration of parameters. In neurologic rehabilitation, the patient's motivation is decisive. The patient, in cooperation from the therapy team, will have to state the goals of his or her rehabilitation. These goals may have to be modified and embedded in a realistic time frame based on consultations between the patient and the therapy team. Only then the patient may be able to summon the necessary endurance to see the rehabilitation through to a successful conclusion.

"For a young man (in neurologic rehabilitation) there can be no better goal than to be able to open a beer can or be able to make a cup of tea."[19,139] With this statement, Barnes and Ward have put the problem of neurologic rehabilitation in a nutshell. The most important player in neurologic rehabilitation is always the patient, for whom rehabilitation is equivalent to extreme hard work.

Note

Exercises should always be as active as possible, by no means passive, and whenever possible, should be performed at the tolerance limit.

Variability on the path to the movement goal plays a fundamental role. First, it helps to avoid boredom and second, it helps to sustainably improve the motor memory. The dosage of the therapy administered is of some significance. Sterr and Freivogel have demonstrated that 6 hours of functional therapy per day leads to better results than 3 hours of therapy.[383]

Therapeutic exercise provides us the opportunity to offer sufficient therapy time even to neurologic patients, indicating that these patients have a chance of achieving motor improvements, which they would not have achieved without the additional training.

5.3 Treatable Neurologic Symptoms in Therapeutic Exercise

Spasticity is defined by Lance[224] as speed-dependent resistance to passive motion. This resistance is comprised of neuronal and biomechanical components (▶Fig. 5.1). Spasticity is a plus symptom of upper motor neuron syndrome. Other plus symptoms include hyperreflexia, clonus, and increased muscle tone. According to Jackson,[197] the complex manifestation of upper motor neuron syndrome includes minus and positive symptoms (▶Fig. 5.2). The minus symptoms include pareses, impairment of selective finger motions, and the inability to perform rapidly alternating movements (▶Table 5.1).[135]

Both plus and minus symptoms occur in a lesion of the upper motor neuron. Spasticity and paresis are two different components of the lesion. Spasticity is not solely responsible for the motor functional problems; these are also due to the concomitant paresis. Spasticity can be reduced by stretching the muscles slowly, stretching while bearing weight (standing, etc.), reciprocal movement (exercise bicycle), or with medication.

However, the reduction in spasticity does not necessarily lead to an improvement of motor skills.[179] Paresis cannot be improved simply by

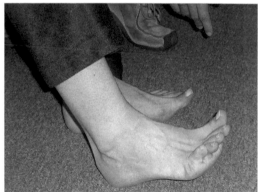

Fig. 5.2 Paresis of the dorsiflexors, compensated with the digital extensors.

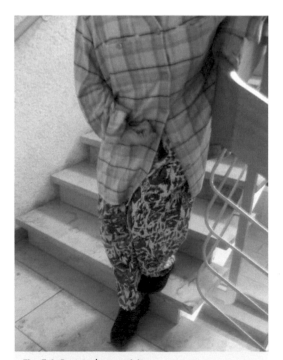

Fig. 5.1 Poststroke spasticity.

Table 5.1 Upper motor neuron syndrome (UMNS)

Plus symptoms	Minus symptoms
• Spasticity	• Paresis, weakness, paralysis
• Clonus	
• Exaggerated reflexes	• Fine motor dysfunction
• Babinski's sign	• Dysdiadochokinesia, slowness
• Associated reactions	
• Mass movements	• Increased effort, rapid exhaustion
	• Limited automatic movements
	• Difficulty in dual tasks

Note: Spasticity is almost invariably associated with paresis of variable severity.

reducing spasticity but only by active repetitive exercise (strength training) and functional activity. Studies have since shown conclusively that repetitive exercise and strength training contribute to the reduction of spasticity and improving the quality of movement (▶Fig. 5.3).[49,382]

5.3.1 Symptom of Spasticity

Recent studies view the development of spasticity as the body's reaction to the weakness or functional deficits caused by the lesion. The primeval principle holds that a living creature must move in order to survive. This is consistent with the notion that from a functional standpoint, walking, standing, and transfer are more readily possible with spasticity than with weakness. This is presumably the reason why the body develops spasticity as a response to CNS lesions.

The severity of the spasticity depends on the location and size of the lesion. Thus, one can expect to find more severe spasticity with a major lesion than with a discrete lesion. With respect to the time frame, one first encounters weakness, whereas spasticity develops only later in the clinical course. This development is readily observable in patients with multiple sclerosis, as the pathophysiology often develops very slowly in multiple sclerosis in contrast to craniocerebral trauma or stroke. From a functional standpoint, weakness is the main problem for patients with moderate to severe multiple sclerosis. Even in a patient with craniocerebral trauma, weakness appears first, followed by development of spasticity within the next few days or weeks. The same applies to a stroke or a paraplegic patient due to spinal shock. Therefore, it is

necessary to initiate and promote activities as early as possible so that the development of spasticity is no longer necessary for functional activities. Thus, active therapy must be initiated as early as possible in the early phase of the disorder; passive forms of therapy must be replaced with active forms.

Cycling trainers are one means of initiating early activity (▶Fig. 5.4). Here, it is important to set a resistance when training both the upper and lower extremities. The motor of a cycling trainer assists the patient's motion but at the same time requires the patient to move actively to stimulate residual function. All cycling trainers provide a function for evaluating the patient's performance after training has been completed. Standing, even in a standing frame, activates the postural muscles (▶Fig. 5.5).

> **Note**
>
> Walking training should be initiated as soon as possible because many muscles are trained in a basal pattern. "Spasticity therapy" does not have the intrinsic purpose of reducing spasticity; useful spasticity therapy should always be combined with functional training (▶Fig. 5.6). Strength training in neurology is helpful, necessary, and reduces spasticity.[138]

Findings in Spasticity

Spasticity can be measured with the Ashworth Scale or the Tardieu Scale (▶Table 5.2). The Ashworth scale or the modifed Ashworth scale (MAS) is widely used by physicians and therapists. The

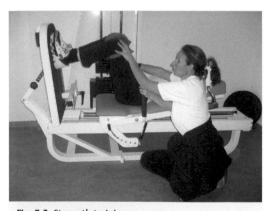

Fig. 5.3 Strength training.

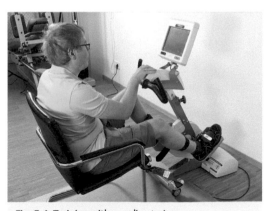

Fig. 5.4 Training with a cycling trainer.

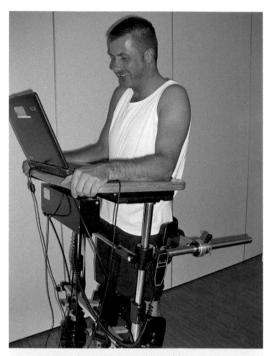

Fig. 5.5 Standing with a standing table.

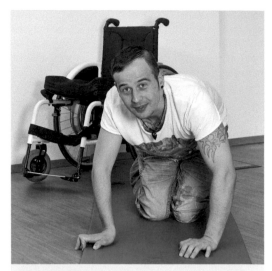

Fig. 5.6 Crawling reduces spasticity while activating functional capacity.

Table 5.2 Ashworth scale

Grade	Severity of spasticity
0	No increase in muscle tone
1	Slight increase in tone
2	More marked increase in muscle tone through most of the range of motion, but affected part(s) easily moved
3	Considerable increase in muscle tone, difficult passive movement
4	Significant increase in muscle tone, difficult rapid passive motion
5	Affected part rigid in flexion or extension

use of MAS is a practical approach but has been repeatedly criticized for its poor-quality criteria. In findings of spasticity, the respective joint of the affected extremity is moved passively; initially slowly, and then rapidly. The resistance is then evaluated accordingly.

The Tardieu scale is currently regarded as the better spasticity scale, as it provides more consideration to the speed-related aspects of spasticity. Patrick and Ada showed in a study that the Tardieu scale was better able to differentiate spasticity from motion impairments or contractures than the MAS (▶Table 5.3).[296]

The Tardieu scale always measures the resistance in passive motion with V1 (as slowly as possible) and V2 (as quickly as possible) making it possible to detect contractures and motion impairments as well.

The clonus test has proven effective as a quick and very simple test of spasticity of the lower extremities, which is able to detect even slight increases in tone. In the clonus test, the patient's forefoot is quickly placed in dorsiflexion, stretching the lower leg. The forefoot is held in this position (▶Fig. 5.7 and ▶Fig. 5.8). The musculature of the lower leg reacts to the rapid stimulation of the muscle spindles with rhythmic contraction, clonus. This test can provide early signs of CNS damage and reveal increased muscle tone. Increased tone begins distally, which increases the sensitivity of the test, such that it is often positive even in the presence of only minor damage. It also lends itself well to comparison of both sides, for example, in a bilaterally affected patient. This is especially important in patients with multiple sclerosis.

5.3.2 Symptom of Paresis

From a functional standpoint, the greatest motor problem in neurologic rehabilitation is the weakness. Unfortunately, weakness is often not the focal point of medical diagnostics and physical therapy findings. The reason that physicians and physical therapists working in neurology often fail to look for weakness is that it does not appear as an obvious primary finding but must be actively sought out.

Yet, even in neurology, weakness can be measured very well with the muscle function test, which can be modified (▶ Table 5.4). The muscle tests are initially performed as passive motion tests, and then the patient is instructed to take

Table 5.3 Tardieu scale

Grade	Description
0	No resistance during passive movement through the full range of motion
1	Slight resistance during passive movement without a definite stop at a certain angle
2	Definite stop at a certain angle that interrupts passive movement but then subsides
3	Exhaustible clonus at a certain angle (lasting less than 10 seconds when the position is maintained)
4	Sustained clonus at a certain angle (lasting more than 10 seconds when the position is maintained)

the weight, at which point, resistance can be provided (▶ Fig. 5.9). It may be necessary to have patients who are only slightly affected to perform some sort of endurance exercise before the muscle test. This would apply to patients who begin to stumble or drag their feet only after having walked for an hour.

Weakness usually occurs in combination with spasticity, and spasticity is more obvious to physical therapists specialized in movement analysis. This implies that the weakness often goes undetected and as a result is not addressed. The physician finds exaggerated reflexes upon examination. For most physicians, exaggerated reflexes reflect spasticity, and for the same reason, physicians no longer look for weakness. Also, no medications are currently available to treat weakness. Thus, weakness in neurologic rehabilitation is the greatest problem; yet, it is often simultaneously the greatest unrecognized problem. Once weakness has been analyzed in everyday situations, treatment is straightforward: intensive strength training and muscular endurance training in the affected muscles. This is where therapeutic exercise plays an indispensable role (▶ Fig. 5.10).

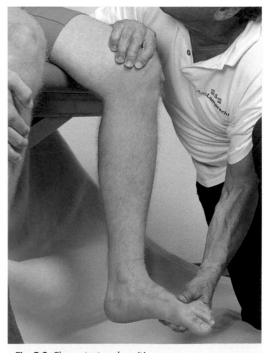

Fig. 5.7 Clonus test starting position.

Fig. 5.8 Clonus test end position.

Table 5.4 Medical Research Council scale (MRC scale) muscle function test

Grade	Test result
0	No muscular activity, complete paralysis
1	Visible and/or palpable contraction without movement
2	Movement is possible when gravity is neutralized
3	Movement against gravity is just barely possible
4	Movement against slight resistance
5	Normal strength

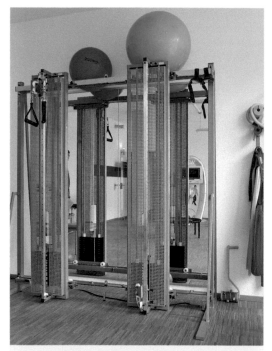

Fig. 5.10 Therapeutic exercise room.

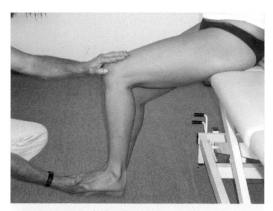

Fig. 5.9 Testing the hip flexors.

5.3.3 Symptom of Ataxia

The literature lacks a single consistent definition of ataxia. According to Patten,[297] ataxia may be understood as an impairment of coordinated motion that is not attributable to paresis or changes in muscle tone, proprioceptive impairments, or sudden involuntary motor sequences.[1] Ataxia is caused by a lesion in the cerebellum or cerebellar pathways. Two of the most common causes of acquired ataxia are multiple sclerosis and craniocerebral trauma. Impaired coordination of the lower extremities due to spinal disorders (posterior column disorders) or peripheral neurogenic disorders (polyneuropathy) are also referred to in the literature as ataxia. This impaired coordination manifests itself as unsteadiness while standing or walking (▶ Fig. 5.11). The main reason for this unsteadiness is the impaired depth perception. Hereditary and acquired disorders associated with degeneration of the cerebellum, and

> **Note**
>
> Ataxia can be tested with:
> - Finger-to-nose test or finger-to-finger test for upper extremity (▶ Fig. 5.12).
> - Heel-to-knee test for lower extremity (▶ Fig. 5.13).
> - Imbalance and gait ataxia can be assessed with the Romberg test or the Unterberger test (▶ Fig. 5.14).
> - Truncal ataxia can be tested in the sitting patient by having the patients shift their weight, although there is no official test for truncal ataxia.

the efferent or afferent pathways can cause ataxic motor impairments.[1]

The patient performs all these tests with eyes open and closed to differentiate cerebellar ataxia from spinal ataxia. If the patient faces significant difficulty in performing the test with eyes closed, depth perception is impaired (afferent pathways to the cerebellum). Patients with multiple sclerosis, in particular, often show spinal ataxia, but so do patients with brainstem trauma or polyneuropathy.

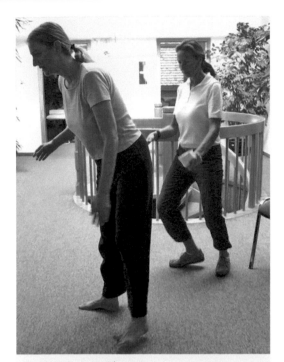

Fig. 5.11 Patient with ataxia.

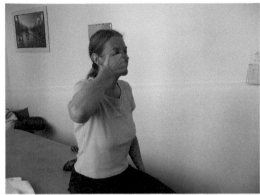

Fig. 5.12 Finger-nose test.

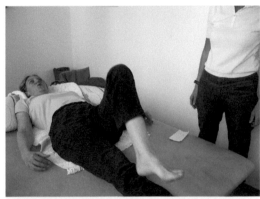

Fig. 5.13 Heel-to-knee test.

Ataxia always occurs on the basis of hypotonia. Therefore, performing strength training is also recommended for ataxia. It is important in ataxia not to train static strength but to perform dynamic strength training. This is because patients with ataxia often attempt to compensate for their ataxia with muscle fixation (▶ Fig. 5.15).

It is easier for patients with ataxia to perform movements against resistance than without resistance. In daily life, these patients often walk with a heavy walker, wear heavy shoes, or wear a heavy jacket or knapsack. Studies have also shown that weights can improve ataxia.[186,61,272] Even wearing a lead vest helped improve truncal stability; however, this led to rapid muscle fatigue (▶ Fig. 5.16).[300]

Patients with ataxia are able to perform rapid movements with much ease. The slower a movement is, the more coordination it requires. The therapist can take advantage of this fact in therapeutic exercise. The rule of thumb for these patients is: More resistance is easier. Reducing the resistance represents shaping or increasing the coordination.

Summary ✔

We can summarize by saying that fast and more resistance is advantageous than slow and less resistance for therapeutic exercise in patients with ataxia.

In daily life, it is easier to set resistance on a cycling trainer than on an exercise bicycle. The cycle ergometers are controlled by power output in watts. This generates fast and little resistance, which in turn, exerts a demand on the cardiovascular system, which is equivalent to slow motion with a lot of resistance. As a general rule, training controlled by power output is not ideal in neurology. As discussed above, weakness is one of the greatest problems that neurologic patients face; neurologic

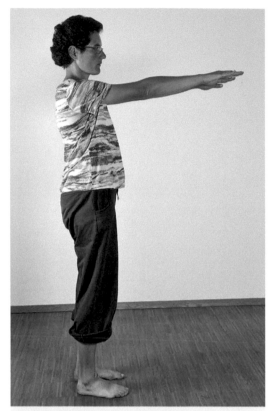

Fig. 5.14 Romberg test.

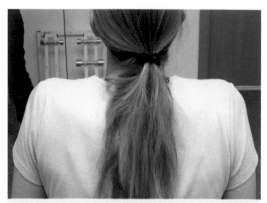

Fig. 5.15 Muscle fixation in ataxia patients.

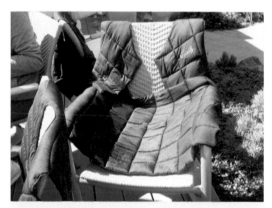

Fig. 5.16 Lead vest.

patients tire relatively quickly and thus become slower. Therefore, it is not a good idea to compound the problem by increasing the resistance.

5.3.4 Symptom of Balance

Neurologic syndromes are associated with loss or impairment of postural control. Postural control generally means the ability to assume an upright body position in space against the force of gravity (▶ Fig. 5.17).[369] In a more specific sense, we can subdivide postural control into static and dynamic components. Static postural control involves balancing the upright position while sitting or standing, whereas dynamic postural control involves balancing a position that is as upright as possible while walking or running.[221]

Balance in Neurologic Rehabilitation

Several factors can impair balance in neurologic patients. Apart from absent or abnormal postural control, both spasticity and paresis can be the cause of balance problems. Yet, even sensory deficits can be responsible for balance problems (Chapter 3). Therefore, it is crucial to obtain precise findings to focus the treatment on patient's specific problems.

Balance is not an independent functional problem; rather, one must determine the causes of the balance impairment when obtaining findings. Balance impairments can be caused by spasticity, paresis, ataxia, or impaired depth perception such as the one that occurs in polyneuropathy. Paresis of the dorsiflexors can occasionally cause extreme balance problems as soon as the patient deviates backward from vertical. Therefore, training must also focus on the causative problem. For example, the dorsiflexors must be activated and strengthened rather than conducting general balance training. Naturally, one could also train the dorsiflexors in a situation where the patient is made to deviate from vertical posteriorly, which would

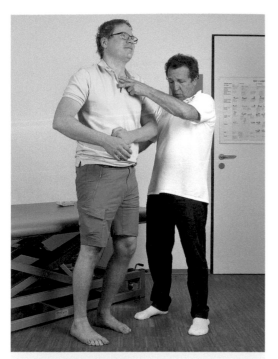

Fig. 5.17 Postural control.

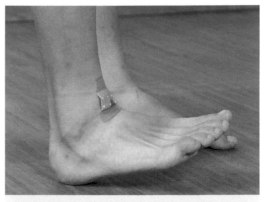

Fig. 5.18 Rhythmic taping: training the dorsiflexors.

train the dorsiflexors, thereby improving the balance problems. However, in addition to this, one would always have to train the dorsiflexors repetitively (▶ Fig. 5.18). This problem is often observed in patients with multiple sclerosis.

If the patients face considerable problems standing with their eyes closed, they must train themselves for it or with incessant rapid redirection of gaze so that they have no opportunity for compensation.

6 Training Equipment in Neurology

6.1 Training Equipment

In this chapter, we present the training equipment that we perceive to be suitable for therapeutic exercise. We will briefly present a few pieces of training equipment that are often observed in fitness studios or therapeutic exercise facilities-intended for orthopaedic and surgical patients but are not specifically suitable for neurologic patients according to our understanding.

We will only briefly mention the robot-assisted training devices that are used primarily in inpatient rehabilitation facilities and less in outpatient centers. Undoubtedly, there are many devices suitable for neurologic therapeutic exercise, which are not discussed here. The development of devices for rehabilitation is very dynamic at the moment with new devices being introduced and existing devices undergoing further development and improvement. It is vital for neurologic therapeutic exercise that the devices can be finely tuned, are easy to use, accessible to persons with disabilities, and allow functional movements.

We have classified the devices according to effect (endurance and strength), although depending on the application of the devices, they can occasionally be utilized for either endurance training or strength training. We are satisfied when users inform us about new devices and when equipment manufacturers further develop their devices so that they can be used for therapeutic exercise in neurology. The important thing is that developers and manufacturers also work together with practitioners and patients to ensure that useful and convenient devices appear on the market.

6.2 Endurance Training

6.2.1 Treadmill

The first treadmill was developed by Nathan Zuntz in 1889. Zuntz was a professor of physiology at the Agricultural College in Berlin. He developed the treadmill to conduct stress studies with horses.

This treadmill had variable speed and inclination and allowed studies under precisely defined, measurable, and reproducible conditions. Zuntz and his coworkers later developed the treadmill to allow measurements in humans as well.

These projects and other work by Zuntz paved the way for what was then the rapidly developing field of sports medicine. Zuntz is also regarded as one of the founders of aviation medicine and a pioneer of high-altitude physiology.

Numerous studies have since led to the widespread acceptance of treadmill and locomotion training as an integral part of the therapy of paraparetic and paraplegic patients and stroke patients with unilaterally paralysis (▶ Fig. 6.1).[173] Initial studies of patients with Parkinson's disease and multiple sclerosis demonstrate greater improvement in many parameters than in gait training without a treadmill.[227] A body weight–supported system (BWST) utilizing a parachute harness or specially developed support beltsallows even severely compromised patients to benefit from treadmill training in the early phase of rehabilitation (▶ Fig. 6.2).

The most important requirement for a treadmill suitable for neurorehabilitation is a very low initial speed, which must be no higher than 0.2 km/h (0.12 mph). Many neurologic and geriatric patients do not tolerate higher speeds when they initiate practice on a treadmill. Speed should be increased in increments of 0.1 km/h (0.06 mph). The option of setting an incline (both uphill and downhill) is also important. A suitable handrail should also be present, ideally one with adjustable height.

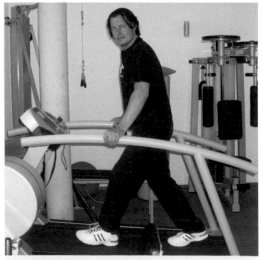

Fig. 6.1 Treadmill training.

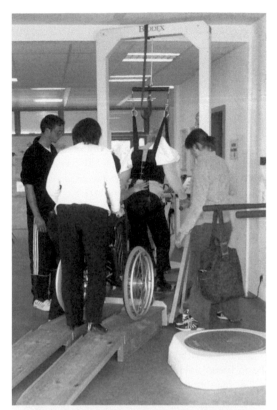

Fig. 6.2 Body weight–supported treadmill (BWST) system.

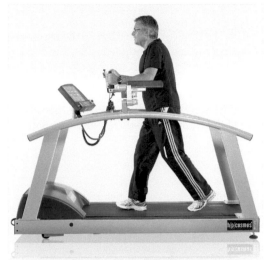

Fig. 6.3 Treadmill with forearm supports. Used with the kind permission of h/p/cosmos sports & medical GmbH, Nussdorf-Traunstein, Germany.

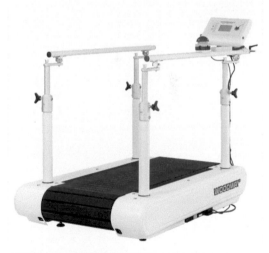

Fig. 6.4 Slat-belt treadmill. Used with the kind permission of Woodway GmbH, Weil am Rhein, Germany.

There are also treadmills with adjustable width handrails. Patient should be able to rest their forearms on special rails (▶ Fig. 6.3).

A smooth suspension system is not necessarily important in neurologic rehabilitation; a slat-belt treadmill is not absolutely necessary. The speed at which patients in neurologic rehabilitation undergo training is not high enough to lead to a float phase while walking. With slat-belt treadmills, it can be difficult to get on the treadmill with the patient, as these treadmills are relatively high because of their design (▶ Fig. 6.4). A ramp is required to bring a wheelchair patient onto a slat-belt treadmill (▶ Fig. 6.5).

If the treadmill includes a built-in ramp, then it must be removed to allow the patient to train independently. The only time when a slat-belt treadmill might be necessary is when it is used in conjunction with certain gait trainers. For example, the LokoHelp was originally designed for use with Woodway treadmills, although it now can be connected to other treadmills. Other gait trainers are also designed to fit only a certain treadmill.

A great many gait trainers are now available on the market, such as Lokomat, LokoHelp, and Pedago. This reflects an increased appreciation of the importance of treadmill training in rehabilitation (▶ Fig. 6.6, ▶ Fig. 6.7).

In one well-designed study, LokoHelp demonstrated an efficacy comparable to that of a treadmill. At the same time, the effort on the part of the therapist was significantly less, and less therapy time was required for gait training.[128]

An exoskeleton or BWST allows even severely disabled patients to benefit from treadmill training in the early phase of rehabilitation. The advantage of gait trainers is that they reduce the physical effort required from the therapist and thus allow a longer training period with a higher number of repetitions for the patient.

The motion sequence of walking on a treadmill is different from overground walking. On a treadmill, the surface moves backward during the stance phase, whereas in overground walking, the weight-bearing leg must move the body forward. This also means that the balance requirements are not identical. Nonetheless, walking on a treadmill is very similar, and it is precisely the receding motion of the surface that triggers the stride reaction. As in four-legged animals, these stride reactions in humans are triggered by the central pattern generators (CPGs) in the spinal cord.[91]

The concept of the CPG postulates the existence of a network of neurons, which can intrinsically, i.e., without an external stimulus, generate alternating activity.[242] Movements, such as walking, running, flying, swimming, chewing, and breathing are generated by these neural networks in the central nervous system (CNS) and adapted to environmental requirements by sensory feedback. Although walking is a voluntary act, it only has to be initiated voluntarily, after which it continues as an independent automatic process. We do no need to think about how we walk because walking

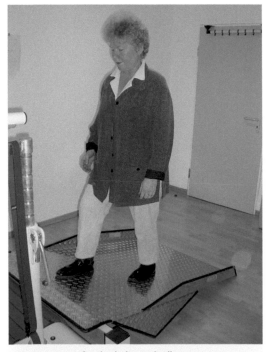

Fig. 6.5 Ramp for slat-belt treadmill.

> **Note**
>
> However, treadmill training can never replace gait training on different surfaces. This reflects the law of identical elements; patients only apply the exercises they have actually practiced to their daily lifes (▶Fig. 6.8, ▶Fig. 6.9, ▶Fig. 6.10).[246]

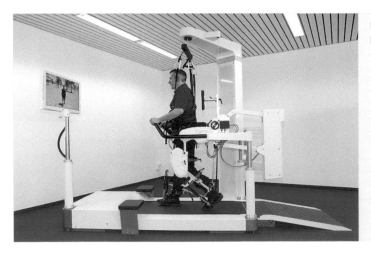

Fig. 6.6 Lokomat. Used with the kind permission of Hocoma, Switzerland.

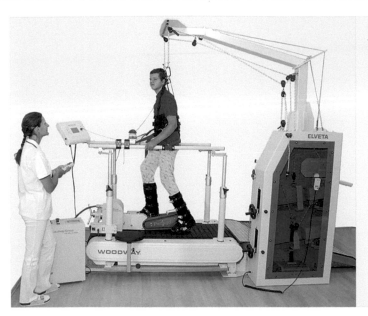

Fig. 6.7 LokoHelp Pedago. Used with the kind permission of www. lokohelp.net.

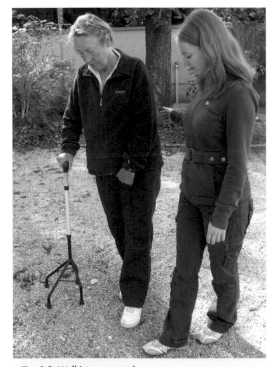

Fig. 6.8 Walking on gravel.

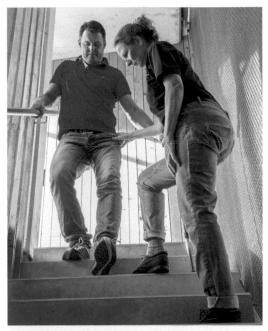

Fig. 6.9 Descending stairs.

is controlled by the spinal circuits.[90] It is assumed that these CPGs, which are thought to be in the spinal cord, are activated each time one foot is placed in front of the other. This activation is irrespective of the way in which the foot is advanced or whether it is advanced actively or passively; the only important thing is that the free leg moves past the weight-bearing leg with each step. Therapists must ensure that this is always the case when passively advancing the feet (▶ Fig. 6.11).

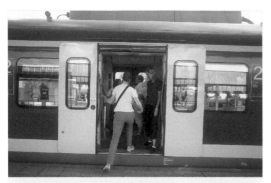

Fig. 6.10 Boarding a commuter train.

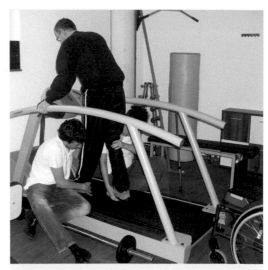

Fig. 6.11 Passively advancing the feet on the treadmill.

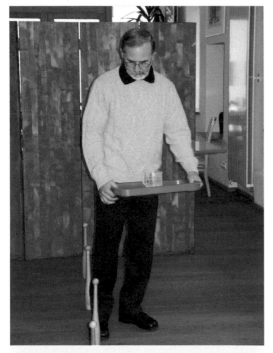

Fig. 6.12 Dual-task training.

Walking is a basal motion pattern that is genetically predetermined and therefore, it is possible to elicit the walking pattern even in severely disabled patients very early in rehabilitation (phase B). This should be exploited intensively in rehabilitation and especially during early rehabilitation. In many patients, the walking pattern can be elicited earlier and easier than simple transfers such as bed to chair or wheelchair to toilet. It may also

be possible to improve the transfer (bed to wheelchair, wheelchair to toilet, and wheelchair to bed) by improving walking. This approach works very well, especially in patients with severe cognitive impairments. It is often not possible to elicit the abstract motion pattern of the transfer in patients with severe cognitive impairments, whereas the gait pattern can be more readily elicited. Therefore, it is better to have the patient practice walking directly on the treadmill with a body weight–support system if practicing the transfer fails. With this approach, walking can often be used to improve standing and transfer. The motor programs for standing and transfer are not as deeply anchored as the walking pattern and therefore are not always easily elicited.

One great advantage of treadmill training over gait training on a surface is the opportunity it offers for dual-task or multi-task training (▶Fig. 6.12). If the patient wants to increase mobility outside the home as well, walking training should be performed in dual-task or multi-task mode.

Definition	[ ]
Dual-task or multi-task training means that patients must also talk, turn their head, carry something, or even perform these things simultaneously in addition to walking.	

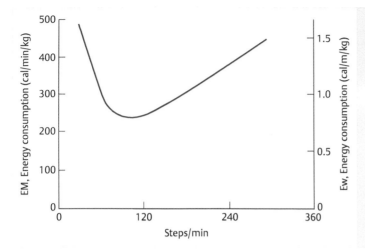

Fig. 6.13 Energy curve for walking at different paces.

Experience has shown that all neurologic patients walk better on the treadmill than overground because they do not have to pay attention to several things simultaneously. The effect is often particularly apparent in patients with Parkinson's disease because the treadmill acts as an external cue for the patient. As dual-task training is particularly difficult in the later phase of Parkinson's disease; these patients should not perform treadmill training primarily in a dual-task situation. This does not mean that dual-task elements cannot be used in training with patients suffering from Parkinson's disease.

It is precisely the receding motion of the treadmill surface that reinforces the stride reaction. In this sense, treadmill training can be regarded as forced-use training of the lower extremities, as the patient is forced to take steps.[161] Many patients have difficulties with the altered motor sequence the first time they use the treadmill or even the second time. Therefore, it is necessary to begin treadmill therapy at a very low speed. Patients get accustomed to the altered motion sequence by the second or third time at the latest but usually within a few minutes. The important thing is to let the patients experience the movement themselves without too many verbal instructions from the therapist; the principles of implicit motor learning apply here, too.

Note that slower walking invariably requires more strength and better balance than faster walking. The most efficient walking takes place at a pace of about 120 steps per minute. The energy required increases exponentially with slower walking (▶ Fig. 6.13). Where patient and therapist can agree to increase the treadmill speed, it often makes the walking easier for the patient. The gait pattern is bound to improve. The same applies to the Pedago or Lokomat; here, too, one should work with a pace approaching the most efficient gait rhythm.

> **Note**
>
> Treadmill training can be used very effectively to train the most important parameters in locomotion and mobility:
> - Walking speed and
> - Walking endurance

Both are important predictors of walking outside the home. Perry et al[301] calculated certain minimum speeds as requirements for walking inside and outside the home:
- Minimum walking speed, 1.1 m/s ≅ 3.96 km/h (3.6 ft/s ≅ 2.46 mph).
- Walking distance of about 500 m (1,640 ft).
- Ability to turn the head while walking.
- Ability to negotiate stairs and curbs.
- Ability to carry objects while walking.

Walking outside the home is among the most important goals of both the patient and neurologic rehabilitation. Walking speed is crucial to mobility and must be trained accordingly. Crossing a street requires a walking speed of about 2.6 km/h or 1.6 mph.[135] The 10 meter walking test is a simple test for measuring walking speed (▶ Table 9.1).

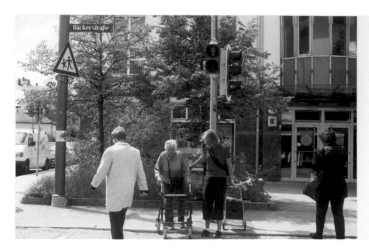

Fig. 6.14 Pedestrian at a traffic light.

Endurance is equally important as walking speed for the patient's mobility.[287] Walking a distance of 300 meters (985 feet) in 11.5 minutes (1.56 km/h or 0.97 mph) is regarded by Lernier–Frankiel et al[232] as a criterion for walking outside the house.[287] This translates into a walking speed of 1.6 km/h or 0.99 mph over a longer distance. International Classification of Functioning, Disability, and Health (ICF, d4501) defines a long distance as 1 km (0.62 miles). The 6-minute walking test is a simple test for measuring walking endurance (▶Table 9.1).

A patient needs both the abilities mentioned above to achieve near normal mobility and thus be in a position to actively participate in activities. Therefore, when formulating the goals of therapy, one should note which of the two is to be trained. If the goal of therapy is walking endurance, then the patient must train for endurance; if it is walking speed, then the patient must train for speed.

Walking endurance is important for the patient to achieve social participation. Walking speed is essential to ensure mobility outside the home, as the switching interval of many pedestrian traffic lights requires a walking speed of 3.6 km/h or 2.2 mph. Such regulations make it difficult for neurologic patients, including many other people who are no longer able to walk very fast, to participate in social life as defined in the ICF. For many patients, this requirement is such a great obstacle that they no longer leave the home and rarely have any social contacts (▶Fig. 6.14).

An ability to walk sufficiently fast and long on a treadmill or walk up and down a hospital corridor or on a smooth surface in a physical therapy facility is enough to ensure meaningful social participation in daily life. According to the law of identical elements described by Majsak,[246] walking, in particular, must be practiced in situations relevant to daily life before one can speak of successful gait rehabilitation. This implies that walking on different types of surfaces, in crowds, and also in rain and snow must also be practiced in therapy. The patient must exercise at the tolerance limit, and therapy planning must observe the principle of shaping.

> **Practical Tip**
>
> **Walking Outside the Home**
> - Minimum walking speed, 1.1 m/s ≅ 3.96 km/h (3.6 ft/s ≅ 2.46 mph).
> - Walking distance of about 500 m (1,640 ft).
> - Ability to turn the head while walking.
> - Negotiating stairs and curbs.
> - Carrying objects.

Genuine mobility also requires the ability to use public transportation (buses and streetcars) and escalators with confidence.[287] Certain health care systems put outpatients at a disadvantage. For example, the framework agreements between the German physiotherapists' associations and health insurance funds are flawed. These agreements stipulate that therapy may only be performed in approved therapy facilities, in the patient's home, or on the premises of social facilities. Such agreements can cause problems with insurance coverage in the event the therapist, for the patient's benefit, conducts gait training outside the premises of the therapy facility and a personal injury occurs.

Summary ✔

To summarize, successful gait rehabilitation cannot be achieved solely with treadmill training. On the contrary, patients require training under various conditions that they encounter in daily life.

Treadmill and Endurance Training

Endurance training on the treadmill is best conducted as interval training. Training intensity depends on the respective clinical syndrome (Chapter 7). Ideally, training should include pulse monitoring. The patient walks as long as possible (Borg scale), ideally remaining within the respective training pulse range, which if possible is measured by an exercise electrocardiogram. Then, the patient takes a break until the pulse has normalized and then continues. The goal is to improve walking endurance and/or cardiovascular endurance.

Treadmill and Strength Training

When using the treadmill for strength training, an uphill incline is utilized to strengthen the calf muscles (▶Fig. 6.15). Patients with hemiplegia and resulting asymmetry can be assisted by placing a long dumbbell or weight bar on their shoulders while they are on the treadmill (▶Fig. 6.16). This aids in achieving symmetry and an upright posture when walking. Walking sideways on the treadmill strengthens the muscles in the stance phase and aids in stabilizing the hips. This exercise may also provide an external focus to correct the foot because abducting the foot to take a step sideways automatically pronates it. Training intensity is increased by elevating the incline of the treadmill and carefully accelerating it (▶Fig. 6.17).

Treadmill and Balance Training

If balance is to be trained on the treadmill, then one must first check to determine what the patient's primary balance problem is. If the patient faces problems with eyes closed, then depth perception or proprioception must be practiced. This

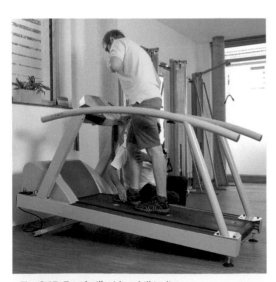

Fig. 6.15 Treadmill with uphill incline.

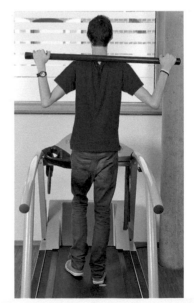

Fig. 6.16 Patient with weight bar on the treadmill.

is performed with the eyes closed (note that this is very difficult on a treadmill) or while shifting the gaze left and right or up and down. Make sure that if the patients do not support themselves, an additional information channel is available that renders the training of proprioception and depth perception significantly less effective. If the

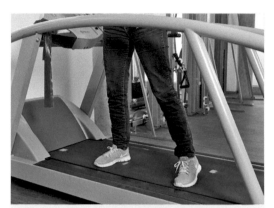

Fig. 6.17 Walking sideways on the treadmill.

patient has problems letting go, putting elastic bands on the handrails to hold on to should often be enough to allow the patient to complete the therapy (▶ Fig. 6.18). Balance is also trained on the treadmill when the patient has to perform other motor or cognitive tasks simultaneously.

Treadmill and Dual-Task Training

Dual tasking or multi tasking can be trained very well on the treadmill. The patient should talk and walk. He or she can catch balls, look for colors or objects in the room, count backward or calculate, or the therapist can throw sandbags on the treadmill that the patient has to avoid. The patient can also carry objects or move them around (▶ Fig. 6.19). The imagination is the limit for devising dual tasks or multi tasks. Here, too, the important thing is for patients to train at their tolerance limit.

Treadmill and Speed Training

The treadmill can be used very well for training walking speed in particular. Speed-dependent

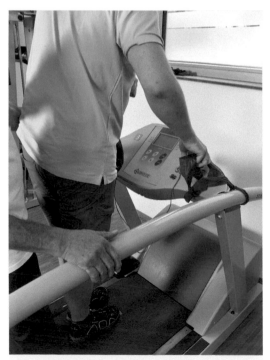

Fig. 6.18 Elastic bands on the treadmill.

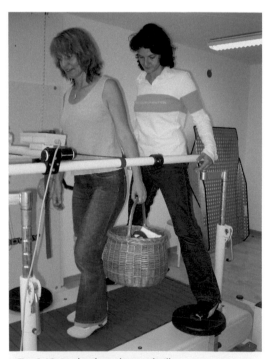

Fig. 6.19 Dual task on the treadmill.

treadmill training (STT) was developed in 1999 and 2000 at the Kreischa rehabilitation clinic and has been the subject of scientific study.[319,320] Using this training system, poststroke patients were able to achieve a much higher walking speed than with other treadmill training methods.[260] Neurologic patients with a diagnosis other than stroke can also benefit from STT.

Structured, speed-based treadmill training always involves pulse monitoring, and the patient is free to abort the training at any time. The patient performs a 10 meter walking test (▶Table 9.1) and then begins with a warm-up phase of about 5 minutes at half the speed achieved in the 10 meter test. Then the speed is increased to the speed achieved during the 10 meter test. The patient maintains this walking speed for 10 seconds. Next, a complete recovery pause is added to allow the patient to approach or return to his resting pulse. If the patient masters the speed on the treadmill with ease and feels confident about it, then the speed is increased 10% at the next attempt. The patient should again maintain this speed for 10 seconds and followed by a pause to return to his resting pulse. If the patient can maintain this speed for 10 seconds without stumbling and feels confident, then the speed is again increased to 10%. In each training session, the speed can be increased up to five times. After this, the patient should spend the remaining training time (approximately 10–15 minutes) walking on the treadmill at a speed of his own choice.

If the patient is unable to maintain the speed for 10 minutes, stumbles, or feels unsure, the speed is reduced to 10% and is only increased later. Following a brief warm-up phase, the next training session begins at the speed last achieved. Each training session lasts about 30 minutes. Speed-dependent treadmill training is performed 3 days a week for a period of 4 weeks. The results demonstrated that all patients could walk completely independently. Maximum walking speed nearly tripled. It was also demonstrated that patients received adequate cardiovascular training without cardiac overload during speed-dependent treadmill training.[260]

The patient has to walk faster when the treadmill runs faster; meaning that the patient must perform forced use training. In walking overground, the patient's motivation is decisive. The patient lacks the external focus, the implicit stimulus to walk faster.

Hamzei et al demonstrated that gait training in the form of constraint-induced movement therapy (CIMT) led to improvement of all gait parameters in chronic stroke patients (▶Fig. 6.20).[161]

Using the Treadmill in Spasticity

In neurologic patients with severe spasticity, walking on the treadmill with or without weight support reduces the spasticity and simultaneously provides functional training for muscle activity in the trunk and lower extremities. Initially, patients can occasionally exhibit a high degree of spasticity. However, this usually subsides after a few steps. As the patient tires and loses strength, the body again responds to this weakness with increased spasticity. This is a sign that the patient should take a break. After a brief pause (1–3 minutes), the patient can resume training.

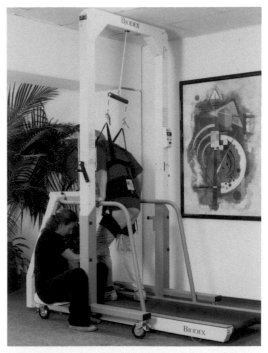

Fig. 6.20 Forced walking with body weight–support system for safety.

Patients can walk uphill, downhill, sideways, or even backward on the treadmill (▶Fig. 6.22).

The German DGN guideline "Rehabilitation of Sensorimotor Impairments" recommends aerobic treadmill training for patients who are already able to walk.[89] The target heart rate (THR) is determined by means of a training paradigm borrowed from cardiologic rehabilitation:

$$THR = (HR_{max} - HR_{rest}) \times 0{:}6 + HR_{rest}$$

HR_{rest} is determined by measuring the pulse for 1 week immediately after waking and then taking the average.

The HR_{max} is determined by exercise ergometry. If this method is not feasible, the following formula is used:

$$HR_{max} = 180 - age$$

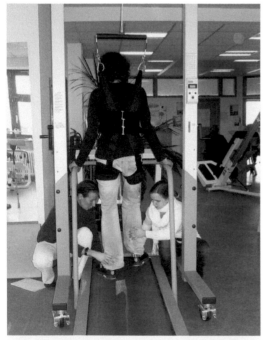

Fig. 6.21 Therapist advancing patient's feet on the treadmill.

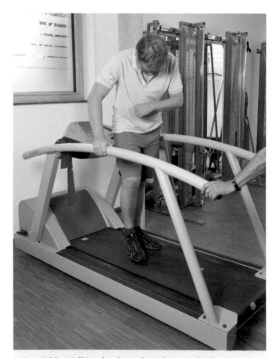

Fig. 6.22 Walking backward on the treadmill.

If the patient is taking β-blockers, the THR is reduced by 15 to 20 beats. Training must include pulse monitoring. The treadmill speed and incline are gradually increased during training to reach the THR. Many treadmills have been designed to accommodate this pulse-controlled training modality so that the optimal heart rate is always reached. Thirty minutes of training per day for a period of 4 weeks is recommended for inpatients and three 45-minute sessions per week for a period of 4 weeks for outpatients.

6.2.2 Cycle Ergometers

Shortly after the invention of the treadmill, Elisée Bouny, the French physiologist, developed the first cycle ergometer in 1896. Today, the cycle ergometer is used in the rehabilitation of all patient groups but especially in cardiovascular rehabilitation.

Good and reasonably priced ergometers are now available for home use (▶ Fig. 6.23). Cycle ergometers are used for endurance or strength training. Modern ergometers are equipped with eddy current brakes. All these ergometers have different programs that allow either constant output (for example 25 watts), an exercise profile, or pulse-controlled exercise. As soon as the patient has sufficient stability in the trunk, he or she can begin training on a cycle ergometer. Some patients can use a recumbent ergometer (▶ Fig. 6.24).

The disadvantage of an ergometer is that the output is determined in watts. This means that as the speed of motion increases, resistance decreases, or conversely, as speed decreases, resistance becomes greater. This is often counterproductive in endurance training for neurologic patients.

Despite this disadvantage, an ergometer can be put to good use in endurance training. Ideally, a physician performs an exercise electrocardiogram beforehand to determine the ideal pulse-controlled training stress. Wherever possible, endurance training on an ergometer should include pulse monitoring. The targets for the training plans are determined by the exercise electrocardiogram or are identical to those in cardiovascular rehabilitation. The same principles apply as in treadmill endurance training. Strength training is possible on an ergometer but is primarily recommended as part of the patient's own home training program. Strength training with a cycling trainer is more effective than with an ergometer.

6.2.3 Upper Body Ergometers

Many neurologic patients, especially wheelchair patients, require good function in the upper extremities and the shoulder and neck region to achieve independence. Patients who are unable to perform endurance training with the lower extremities can do this with an upper body

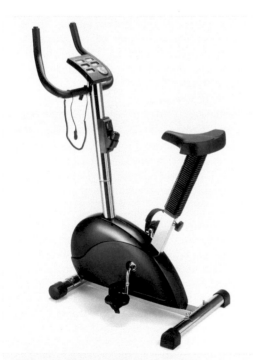

Fig. 6.23 Cycle ergometer for home use.

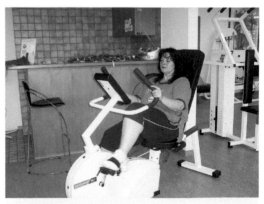

Fig. 6.24 Recumbent ergometer.

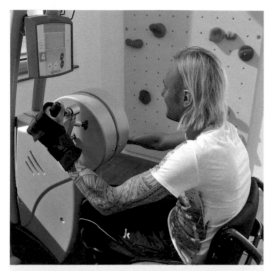

Fig. 6.25 Upper body ergometer.

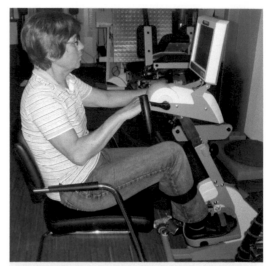

Fig. 6.26 Patient with multiple sclerosis training with a cycling trainer.

ergometer (▶Fig. 6.25). Strength training for the upper extremities and the shoulder girdle is necessary, as autonomous transfer is only possible with good function in the upper extremities.

Training Controlled by Power Output

As a general rule, there is little need for training controlled by power output in watts in neurology. Training controlled by power output was developed for cardiovascular patients. In this training, the resistance is increased when the speed decreases to achieve a constant load on the cardiovascular system. In neurology, this is often counterproductive, as in many neurologic patients, the muscles tire initially, yet require unchanging resistance for endurance training. Such training is possible with a cycling trainer (Chapter 6.2.5). Mostert and Kesselring[274] reported in a study that in patients with multiple sclerosis, fatigue was improved by 30 minutes of bicycle endurance exercise with an individual load of 5 days a week over a period of 4 weeks. Pfitzner et al[305] also demonstrated that patients with multiple sclerosis who underwent 12 sessions (45 minutes each) of endurance training with a cycle ergometer over a period of 2 weeks displayed significant improvement in fatigue according to the Modified Fatigue Impact Scale (MFIS) and the Expanded Disability Status Scale (EDSS, ▶Fig. 6.26).

6.2.4 Elliptical Trainers

The elliptical trainer is so called because of its drive system. With its two arm levers, it allows a pattern of motion similar to that of Nordic walking (▶Fig. 6.27). A study by Marshall et al found that it was not possible to use the watt output on the unit's monitor to control training on the elliptical trainer. The actual physical output generated by using the elliptical trainer is unknown. For this reason, the manufacturers recommend basing exercise regimes on heart rate.[251]

> **Note**
>
> Elliptical trainers have the advantage that the motion sequence is familiar, and that the simultaneous motion of both arms and legs provides support for the weaker extremities.

The cardiostrong elliptical cross trainer, EX90, has advantages over other elliptical trainers in that it permits access from the rear and has locking pedal arms. This makes it more convenient for severely impaired patients to get on the trainer (▶Fig. 6.28).

The stride length can also be adjusted. The elliptical trainers are suitable for endurance training if they can be used in a pulse-controlled mode. However, planned training is nearly impossible given that the load cannot be set precisely. The NuStep

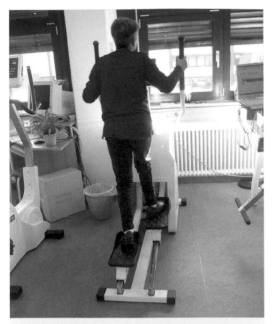

Fig. 6.27 Neurologic patient on an elliptical trainer.

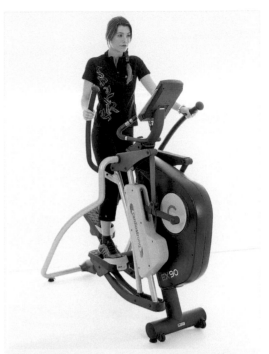

Fig. 6.28 Elliptical cross trainer, EX90. Used with the kind permission of Sport-Tiedje GmbH, Schleswig, Germany.

is a new development among elliptical trainers. It is a combination of recumbent cycle ergometer, elliptical trainer, and stepper (▶ Fig. 6.29). It can be used for full-body motion and for training only the upper body or the legs. It is also recommended for geriatric patients or severely impaired neurologic patients who are unable to use an elliptical trainer in a standing position. The intelligent design makes it very convenient for users to get on the NuStep, even severely impaired patients. The seat can be rotated 360 degrees, and the arm and leg levers are individually adjustable, as is a fixation system for the arms and legs. The disadvantage with the NuStep is the power output control in watts; it is not possible to train without it.

6.2.5 Cycling Trainers

Cycling trainers are available from the manufacturer, Reck (MOTOmed) or Medica (Theravital). The advantage of cycling trainers over ergometers is that they can be precisely adjusted with or without power output control in watts (▶ Fig. 6.30).

An important feature for severely impaired patients in particular is that the motion can be assisted by an electric motor, thus allowing passive motion as well. In spite of this, it is important for the therapist to always set a slight resistance

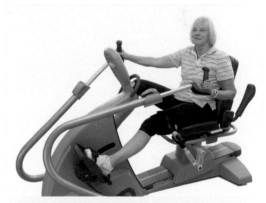

Fig. 6.29 NuStep. Used with the kind permission of Physioaspect Linke GmbH, Freiburg, Germany.

not only to allow passive motion and reduction in spasticity but also to activate and strengthen the muscles. Reciprocal motion helps to regulate muscle tone in the presence of hypertonia.

Visual control and comparison of the left and right sides are also possible with cycling trainers (▶ Fig. 6.31). Symmetrical training is crucial,

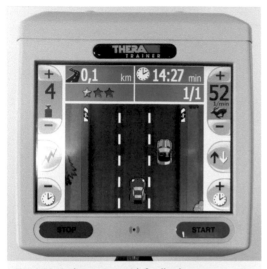

Fig. 6.30 Cycling trainer with feedback.

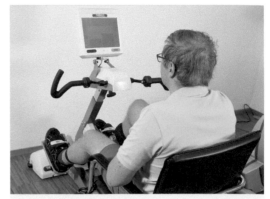

Fig. 6.31 Symmetry training with a cycling trainer.

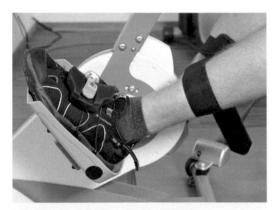

Fig. 6.32 Foot binding on a cycling trainer.

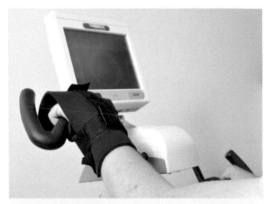

Fig. 6.33 Glove for paretic hand.

especially in patients with hemiplegia or asymmetry, as without this visual control, there is the danger that the patient may perform the main activity with the stronger leg. Therefore, even with a cycling trainer, one should be alert to patients pushing and pulling only with one leg and not exercising the weaker leg.

To reduce the chance of giving patients the illusion of symmetry when training the lower extremities, the foot binding on the less affected side should be left open (▶Fig. 6.32). This symmetry training is also necessary for the upper extremity.

Gloves with velcro closures for arm paresis are available for cycling trainers (▶Fig. 6.33) as are the armrests that allow patients with arm or hand paresis to use the cycling trainer without pain (▶Fig. 6.34).

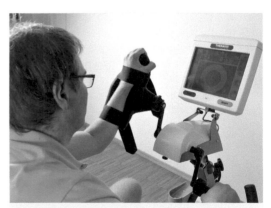

Fig. 6.34 Armrest for cycling trainer.

> **Note**
>
> This same rule applies to the upper extremity. Even motor-assisted movement of the extremity is always better than no movement.

If the patient is in pain, therapist should know the best way to neutralize it. For example, shoulder pain can be controlled with an appropriate bandage such as Neurexa by Otto Bock or a splint, by changing the initial position, or by taping (▶ Fig. 6.35).[281]

A cycling trainer should always offer an opportunity to train both the upper and lower extremities. Even for a neurologic patient who has no problems with the arms, it is extremely important to strengthen the shoulder girdle if the patient uses crutches or a walker or sits on a wheelchair. A cycling trainer for the lower extremities may be sufficient only for those patients who do not require walking aids and have no problems in the shoulder girdle.

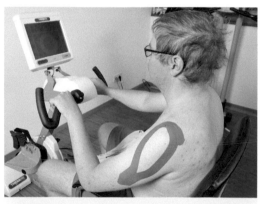

Fig. 6.35 Shoulder tape.

Patients with spasticity can achieve normalized muscle tone with a cycling trainer while simultaneously activating and strengthening their muscles. The reciprocal motion in a cycling trainer quickly and effectively normalizes muscle tone. If a resistance is set, it also achieves functional activation of the musculature.

Patients with ataxia also benefit from training on a cycling trainer. Patients with ataxia usually train with relatively strong resistance and a high speed. Increasing the requirement for patients with ataxia means slower speeds with less resistance.

> **Practical Tip**
>
> **Games**
>
> In developing the new generation of cycling trainers, design engineers have appreciated the importance of visual control and feedback in neurologic and geriatric rehabilitation (▶ Fig. 6.36). Cycling trainers now offer a large number of motion games that even allow two or more players to play against each other.

The reciprocal motions produced when training the arms and legs with the cycling trainer reduce the spasticity as well as provide functional strength and endurance training.

Cycling trainers can also be used by severely impaired patients, as they allow both active and passive motion. The technology is now so advanced that setting training parameters is very easy. Modern cycling trainers offer many different forms of training, some of which are:

- Active training: Training with the patient's own muscle strength (like on a cycle ergometer).

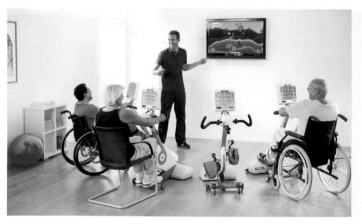

Fig. 6.36 Group training with cycling trainers. Used with the kind permission of medica Medizintechnik GmbH, Hochdorf, Germany.

- Assisted training: Training with residual muscle strength (motor assistance compensates for lack of intrinsic activity).
- Passive training: Training without residual muscle strength (the motor moves the arms or legs).
- Symmetry training: Training for right or left deficits in the legs (such as in stroke patients).

In patients with hemiparesis, the foot should not be immobilized, as pulling with the normal leg can give the illusion of symmetry. For this reason, the better leg should not be immobilized. One can also minimize favoring the normal leg by placing a ping pong ball between the heel and the heel ridge.

All cycling trainers have a spasticity detection function. When a spastic episode occurs, the cycling trainer stops, reverses the direction of motion to resolve the spasticity, and then begins the motion again.

The important thing is that patients regularly train on their own and for a longer period of time. Dobke et al[95] demonstrated that the stroke patients benefit from regular training at home on a cycling trainer (at least twice daily for 10 minutes over 4 months) in terms of improved mobility, quality of life, and performance.

In another study, Ridgel et al[336] demonstrated that training with a cycling trainer at 90 rpm can improve rigor, tremor, and akinesia in patients with Parkinson's disease (MOTOmed viva2 Parkinson, manufactured by Reck). Laupheimer et al also demonstrated that 40 minutes of daily training for the legs with the MOTOmed viva2 at 90 rpm over 10 weeks not only improved gait in patients with Parkinson's disease, but also improved the fine motor function of the hand (▶Fig. 6.37).[228]

6.2.6 Steppers

The stepper simulates climbing stairs (▶Fig. 6.38). The motion sequence is easy to learn; the same principles apply to controlling training as with the elliptical trainer, signifying that endurance training on a stepper should always include pulse monitoring.[251]

Training with a stepper definitely increases the strength in the lower extremities. However, training can only be controlled according to the Borg scale. The HapticWalker is a further development of the stepper. It can be used to train climbing stairs and walking even in early rehabilitation and in severely impaired patients (▶Fig. 6.39). The HapticWalker was originally a prototype developed in cooperation with the Fraunhofer Institute for Production Systems and Design Technology IPK by the working group under Prof. S. Hesse, who later developed the G-EO along with Reha Technologies, Switzerland. Hesse et al demonstrated the efficacy

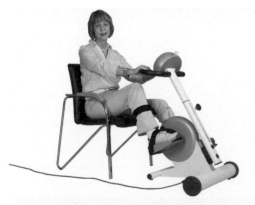

Fig. 6.37 MOTOmed viva2 Parkinson. Used with the kind permission of RECK-Technik GmbH & Co. KG, Betzenweiler, Germany.

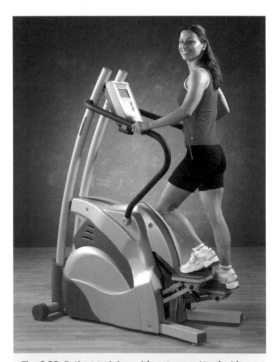

Fig. 6.38 Patient training with a stepper. Used with the kind permission of ERGO-FIT GmbH & Co. KG, Pirmasens, Germany.

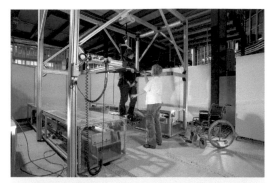

Fig. 6.39 HapticWalker. Used with the kind permission of Fraunhofer Institute for Production Systems and Design Technology IPK, Norbert Michalke.

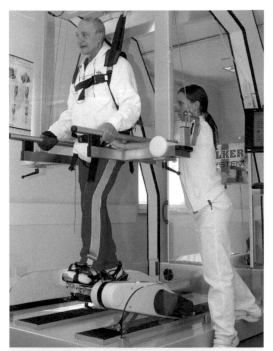

Fig. 6.40 G-EO System Evolution. Used with the kind permission of Reha Technologies 2010 G-EO Systems.

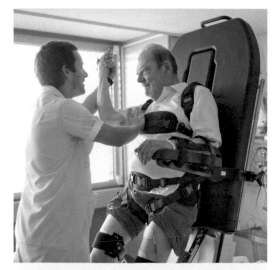

Fig. 6.41 Erigo. Used with the kind permission of Hocoma, Volketswil, Switzerland.

circulatory training. This physiologic cyclic leg motion can be adjusted to each individual patient as required and minimizes the risk of a drop in the blood pressure. The Erigo functional electrical stimulation (FES) can further improve blood circulation in the lower extremities. The stimulation by the Erigo FES is completely synchronized with the cyclic leg motion. The therapist can easily control up to eight FES channels via Erigo's touchscreen to match them to the patient's requirements and ability.[64]

of the G-EO in two studies (▶ Fig. 6.40).[175,177] The G-EO underwent further development and is now available in several different versions. The G-EO System Evolution now implements many options for gait training: walking on a level surface, partial movements, climbing stairs, descending stairs, intelligent control, and visual scenarios.

The Erigo was developed by the Hocoma Company to accustom patients to the upright position even during early rehabilitation (▶ Fig. 6.41). The Erigo is continuously adjustable and can bring the patient from a supine position into a position of 80 degrees. The patient experiences intensive motion therapy with cyclic loading and relief of the lower extremities and at the same time very effective

6.3 Strength Training

Over the last few years, increasing number of studies have been conducted on the subject of strength training for neurologic patients. It was once commonly thought that strength training leads to increased spasticity. Indeed, this opinion is occasionally espoused even today. However, to date, not a single study has ever demonstrated that strength training increases spasticity. On the contrary, all studies have shown that strength training leads to a reduction in spasticity and an improvement in the activities of daily life. Pak et al[292] evaluated the studies on strength training in a review and precisely concluded the same. Frommelt[138] deduced from this study that voluntary motor action triumphs over spasticity. Frommelt[138] also described the parameters Pak and Patten recommended for strength training for poststroke patients with hemiparesis (▶ Table 6.1).

We would like the readers to refer to Chapter 7 for information about strength training in various clinical pictures.

6.3.1 Leg Press

Leg presses in neurologic rehabilitation should be adjusted so that the patients train in a position nearly corresponding to the physiologic position when walking (▶ Fig. 6.42). This means that the patient should be positioned as flat as possible on the leg press so that knee extension can be practiced with the hip in near maximum extension.

Concentric and eccentric training is possible with the leg press. Muscular endurance and maximum strength are the goals of training on the leg press. In terms of mobility skills for the patient, this piece of equipment primarily helps to develop muscular endurance. To be genuinely mobile, the patient must develop sufficient strength and muscular endurance to be able to climb and descend several flights of stairs. Climbing or descending stairs requires the ability to move our body concentrically and eccentrically with one leg several times (▶ Fig. 6.43).

Knee extension should be practiced on soft foot pads in training to improve proprioception (▶ Fig. 6.44). Special attention should be given to properly aligning the axis of the leg. The patient must be instructed to hold the leg in external rotation, as training will not be effective if the thigh is internally rotated. Placing a soft ball between patient's knees and instructing the patient not to press it together is a helpful aid. Alternatively, a

Table 6.1 Strength training in neurologic patients

Training parameters	Recommendation
Intensity of resistance in strength training	60–80% of the maximum resistance achieved in one repetition
Type of exercises	Increase not only strength but also speed
Number of repetitions	8–10, at most 12 per exercise task
Number of exercise tasks	3 per training hour with 8–10 repetitions each
Number of training sessions per week	At least 3
Duration of training	6–12 weeks
Medical contraindications	Before training clinical examination by internist or cardiologist with exercise ECG where indicated
Type of training	Either on equipment or with gait training

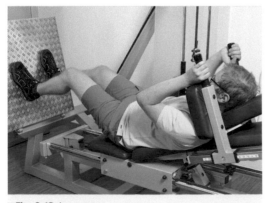

Fig. 6.42 Leg press.

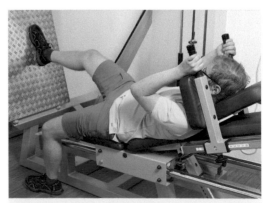

Fig. 6.43 Leg press with one leg.

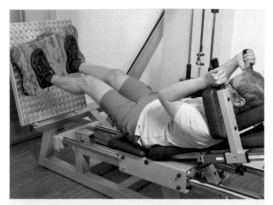

Fig. 6.44 Leg press with a mobile pad.

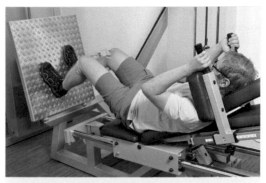

Fig. 6.45 Leg press with the patient maintaining proper axial alignment of the legs.

light elastic band can be placed around the knee. The patient is then instructed to maintain slight tension on this elastic band (▶Fig. 6.45).

Neurologic patients, especially those with asymmetrical strength deficits, must practice with only one leg. Stroke patients, for example, would always favor the unaffected side so that the strength training would not be effective for the affected side. Nearly all neurologic patients exhibit asymmetrical findings; the weaker side requires more intensive training. The patient must be able to repeat the movement 8 to 10 times.

6.3.2 Climbing Wall

A climbing wall is an ideal piece of equipment for functional strength training and for knee extension (Chapter 6.6).

6.3.3 Butterfly Reverse

The butterfly apparatus is one of the preferred strength training devices in fitness centers, as it can train the pectoralis. In neurologic rehabilitation, the pectoralis tends to be hypertonic. Far more important for activities of daily life are the antagonists of the pectoralis, namely the rhomboideus muscles and the other muscles of the back in the region of the upper thoracic spine and in the shoulder and neck region. These posterior muscle groups can be trained very well with the butterfly reverse unit (▶Fig. 6.46).

Training focuses on activating the scapular muscles. The weights that are applied should be enough to allow the patient to perform the motion slowly and evenly. The motion should be initiated by the scapular muscles. Training intensity can be

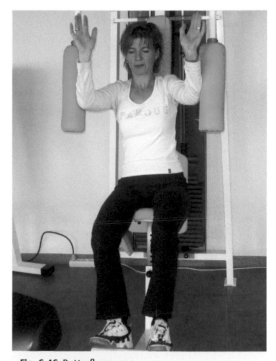

Fig. 6.46 Butterfly reverse.

increased by increasing the repetitions or series before increasing the weight.

6.3.4 Vertical Lat-Pull Machine

Both the anterior and posterior trunk muscles can be trained with the lat-pull machine (▶Fig. 6.47). To train on it, patients must have sufficient stability in the trunk to sit upright. When the vertical axis lies in front of the center of gravity, the anterior muscles are trained; when the vertical axis lies behind the center of gravity, the posterior muscles are trained (▶Fig. 6.48). Trunk training is better when the weights to be lifted are light, as training is not intended to strengthen the arms.

6.3.5 Weight Bars

Weight bars are excellent aids that should be available in every physical therapy facility. As these are relatively inexpensive, patients can also purchase them for use at home.

Weight bars are suitable for many exercises. Their large diameter makes them easier for most patients to handle than long barbells (▶Fig. 6.49). Weight bars are available in different weights. Carrying a weight bar on the shoulders while walking, stimulates a patient to assume an upright posture.

Using weight bars and long barbells:
- Weight bars or long barbells on the trunk improves the patient's upright posture; it also improves the symmetry where truncal asymmetry is present.

- Walking on the treadmill with weight bars or long barbells improves the truncal symmetry (▶Fig. 6.50). The important thing is to place sufficient weight on the shoulders.
- In the presence of truncal asymmetry, patients can also jump with weight bars or long barbells to improve their overall strength (▶Fig. 6.51).
- They can also perform deep knee bends or stand on their toes in the stance phase to increase strength (▶Fig. 6.52).

6.3.6 Long Barbell

Even without weights, long barbells are too heavy and hard to handle for many neurologic patients (▶Fig. 6.53).

6.3.7 Short Barbell

Short barbells can be put to good use with many neurologic patients for a great number of exercises, although they only train individual muscle groups.

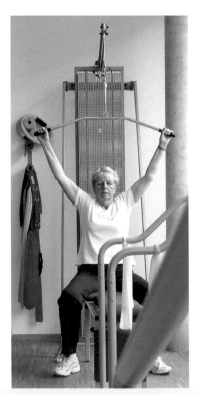

Fig. 6.47 Lat-pull machine.

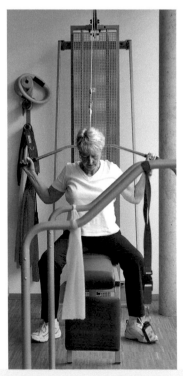

Fig. 6.48 Training posterior muscles on the lat-pull machine.

6.3.8 Knee Extensors and Flexors

We feel that training with a knee curl machine in a sitting position from a 90-degree flexion is not suitable for neurologic patients. Many of these patients have shortened hamstrings, which cause a reactive inhibition of the knee extensors during active knee extension in a sitting position (▶Fig. 6.54). This inhibition renders knee extensor training largely ineffective. Patients with well-stretched hamstrings can practice effectively on a knee curl machine. If the patient can train the knee flexors lying supine on a leg curl machine (▶Fig. 6.55), the machine may serve as an alternative to the leg press, although it may be considerably less effective for knee extension.

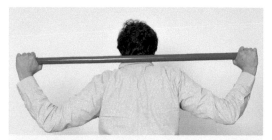

Fig. 6.49 Weight bar.

6.4 Balance Training

Because of the small load-bearing area and the high center of gravity, both standing and walking in an upright position are naturally unstable postures. Many factors can influence or disturb this precarious balance. Patients with neurologic disorders, in particular, can have balance problems for a wide variety of reasons. Balance training must consider the causes to be suitable and effective.

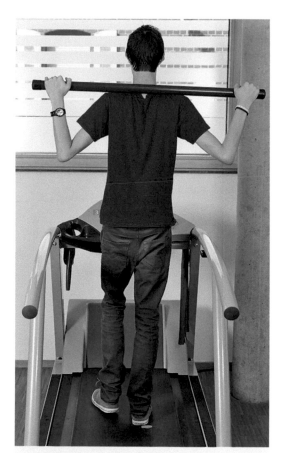

Fig. 6.50 Patient on the treadmill with weight bar to improve symmetry.

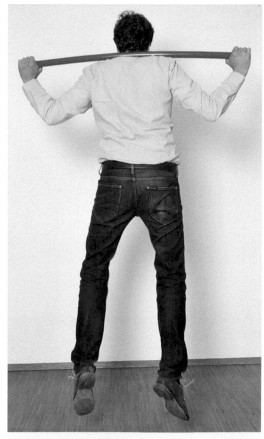

Fig. 6.51 Jumping with the weight bar.

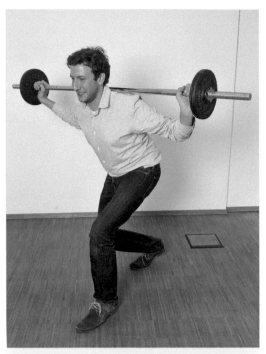

Fig. 6.52 Deep knee bends with the long barbell.

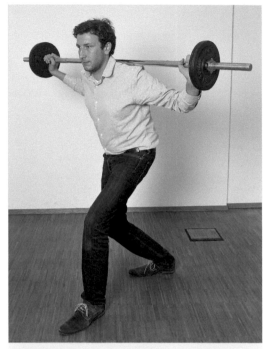

Fig. 6.53 Long barbell.

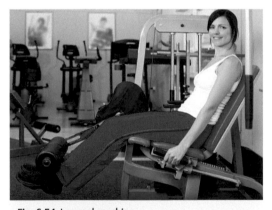

Fig. 6.54 Leg curl machine.

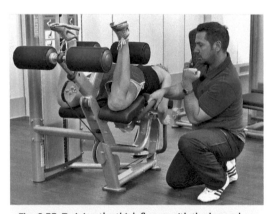

Fig. 6.55 Training the thigh flexors with the leg curl machine.

Reasons for balance problems in neurologic patients can include:
- Impaired depth perception
- Sensory deficits
- Weakness in the foot dorsiflexors when the body's center of gravity is shifted posteriorly
- Diplopia
- Spasticity
- Paresis

6.4.1 Balance Trainers

The balance trainer makes it possible for persons who are partially or completely compromised to stand safely and dynamically (▶ Fig. 6.56). The balance trainer can be individually adjusted, allowing each patient to effectively train balance as well as strength in the trunk and legs. Balance training can

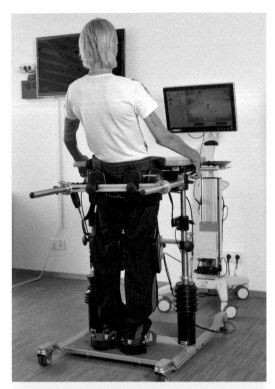

Fig. 6.56 Dynamic balance trainer.

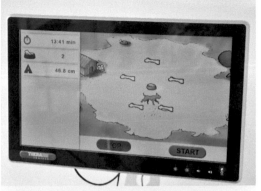

Fig. 6.57 Visual feedback on a dynamic balance trainer.

The adjustable resistance spring of the balance trainer has several different settings that allow patients to train either mobility or strength, depending on how high the resistance is set. A low-resistance setting is best for training balance, whereas a high setting lays more emphasis on strength (▶Fig. 6.58).

6.4.2 SpaceCurl

The SpaceCurl is a triaxial training and therapy machine that works like a gyroscope. Users stand upright in the machine and can move themselves in all three planes by moving or shifting their weight (▶Fig. 6.59). The first machines of this type were developed in Germany to train pilots. NASA uses similar equipment for training astronauts. In medicine, the SpaceCurl is used as a therapy device primarily for three-dimensional functional training of the spine and only rarely in the treatment of neurologic disorders. Motion in the SpaceCurl strengthens the muscles and trains, improves, or restores proprioception and coordination.

The patient is secured in the system by a foot fixation system and pelvic cushions. Severely affected patients who are unable to stand without support can use the SpaceCurl with the aid of a special attachment that holds the patient's knees in extension. Enabling one individual ring initially allows only one movement, back and forth, by placing weight on the heel or forefoot, respectively. Enabling the second ring adds the right–left motion component.

Motion in this plane only occurs if the patient shifts his or her weight. Raising the body's center

be conducted not only in the coronal plane but also in the sagittal plane.

Targeted therapy is possible with a balance trainer as well, especially when used in combination with a monitor that provides visual feedback (▶Fig. 6.57). With the appropriate software and a motion sensor, patients can play different games in which they control the figures by shifting their weight. The games are an effective way to motivate patients and even have them train on their own.

The patient's range of motion to the left and right and forward and backward must be determined before beginning the balance training. These values are then entered as maximum values for the motion, allowing even patients with a very small range of motion to perform all their motion tasks in the balance trainer. The system automatically stores all values, both measured and training values, immediately. This allows very thorough documentation, making it easy to quickly program an increasing degree of difficulty. The visual presets can be used for specific training of patients with pusher syndrome or neglect.

of gravity with the foot platform can shift the focus of training between balance and strength.

The patient in the SpaceCurl receives immediate vestibular and optical feedback. The disadvantage of the SpaceCurl is that patients need assistance to get in and out of the machine. Also, it is not possible for patients to enable the individual planes of motion themselves. Nonetheless, the SpaceCurl is an ideal training machine for neurologic patients. Stroke patients can be specifically instructed to use their affected side. The position of the rings clearly shows the patients' ability to successfully perform this.

Depending on the therapist's instructions, the patient can also train the dorsiflexors by shifting the body's center of gravity slightly backward. This elicits a response from the entire anterior chain, especially the tibialis anterior to maintain the posture. All this occurs under conditions resembling those of daily life and with an external focus, thus in a manner consistent with the principles of motor learning (Chapter 5.2).

Patients with ataxia can practice shifting their weight in a controlled, coordinated manner in the SpaceCurl (▶ Fig. 6.60). If patients stand in the SpaceCurl with a low center of gravity, they must overcome greater resistance to shift their weight. For patients with ataxia, this is easier than without resistance. If the therapist wants to increase the requirements for the ataxia patient (shaping), he or she raises the body's center of gravity. Even slight changes in the load will lead to a large excursion in the movement.

A similar approach is possible for patients with pusher syndrome, forcing the patient to immediately develop a solution strategy from the vestibular and visual feedback (▶ Fig. 6.61). As their feet are fixed, patients are in a controlled situation and receive immediate visual and vestibular feedback about their body's center of gravity.

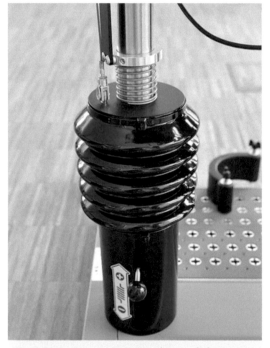

Fig. 6.58 Resistance spring on a dynamic balance trainer.

> **Note**
>
> The great advantage of training with the Space-Curl is, in addition to optimal conditions for motor learning (external focus and feedback), the therapist does not have to work on the patient by pulling or pushing. Instead, the patient receives immediate feedback.

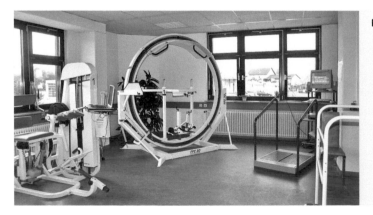

Fig. 6.59 SpaceCurl.

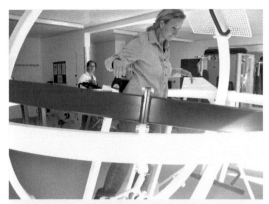

Fig. 6.60 SpaceCurl, right and left movement.

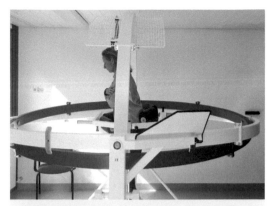

Fig. 6.61 SpaceCurl, visual feedback from the rings.

6.4.3 Physiomat

The Physiomat is a computerized holistic testing and training machine that can be used to train balance, coordination, concentration, and strength. The Physiomat resembles a three-dimensional therapy gyroscope with adjustable resistance and visual feedback. A vibrator plate can also be used, providing continuously adjustable vibration that can be readily activated or deactivated. The Physiomat has many exercise programs that provide the patient different types of tasks as games, which help to increase the patient's motivation. The Physiomat can also document and visualize the patient's progress in training. It can also be fitted with an adapter for the arms and for use by a seated patient.

6.4.4 Posturomed

The Posturomed is a training machine with an unstable standing surface for proprioceptive and sensorimotor training. Müller et al[278] developed a means of measuring the success of sensorimotor training with the Posturomed. The Posturomed was developed primarily as a training device for patients with hip and knee injuries and/or surgery. Even neurologic patients can readily perform balance training on the Posturomed.

A railing on three sides of the Posturomed ensures patient safety. Fastening therabands to the railing can offer patients a semiconstrained option that avoids the external sensory input of grasping the railing.

The Posturomed may be used for a wide variety of therapeutic applications. Used in combination with a pad, the Posturomed can be a genuine challenge even for well-rehabilitated patients. Patients can train balance in dual tasks, such as juggling

two or more balls, practicing with eyes open or closed, and practicing while turning the head back and forth or moving it up and down.

On the Posturomed, too, it is important for patients to train at their tolerance limit. The Posturomed should be used not only for training balance but also strength and dexterity. For example, while standing on one or two pads on the Posturomed, the patient can take a step down and return to the initial position immediately after making contact with the floor (▶Fig. 6.62 and ▶Fig. 6.63). Very well-rehabilitated patients can also jump while on the Posturomed and then stabilize it as quickly as possible in the rest position (▶Fig. 6.64).

6.4.5 Various Pads

Many manufacturers supply pads whose compressive strength can vary greatly. These pads can be used for balance tasks and to enhance the patient's coordination and concentration skills. The disadvantage of these pads is that patients get used to them very quickly. This effect can be reduced if the therapist repeatedly requires the patient to perform a number of different tasks in a randomized order.

6.4.6 Terrasensa

Terrasensa is a textured floor tile that can be extended as desired. Thus, it offers a high degree of variability for training the neuromuscular sensorimotor system. In contrast to other soft floor mats, there is no familiarization effect with Terrasensa, as the irregularities of the floor tiles produces different sensory input each time. The tiles have different surface textures. Terrasensa tiles can be combined very well with other devices for sensorimotor training. They may be used in dual-task training with

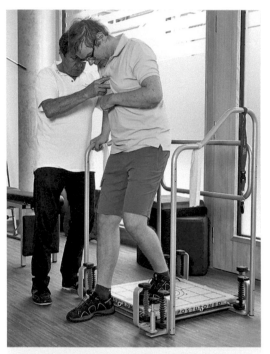

Fig. 6.62 Posturomed, step starting position.

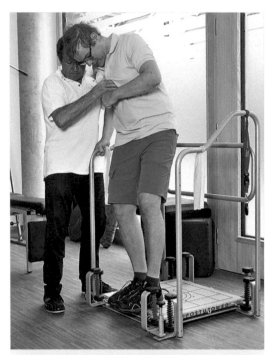

Fig. 6.63 Posturomed, step end position.

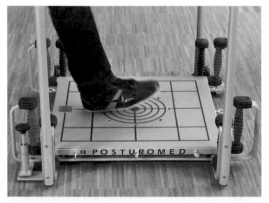

Fig. 6.64 Jumping on the Posturomed.

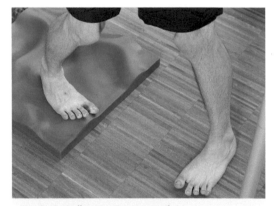

Fig. 6.65 Walking on Terrasensa tiles.

juggling or walking forward, backward, or sideways (▶Fig. 6.65, ▶Fig. 6.66, ▶Fig. 6.67).

6.4.7 Measurement, Therapy, Documentation

The MTD (measurement, therapy, documentation) device offers a large number of measurement and training options (▶Fig. 6.68 and ▶Fig. 6.69). The patient stands on two sturdy measuring plates, suggesting that the majority of neurologic patients

can use the MTD. Patients must be able to stand on their own with support at least briefly.

Advantages of this unit include its broad spectrum of applications and precise tests. The device is also very popular among patients of all age groups. It strengthens patients' ambition and motivation by presenting them with various tasks in the form of games. It would be helpful if the developers could expand the range of therapeutic games that patients can play with the MTD.

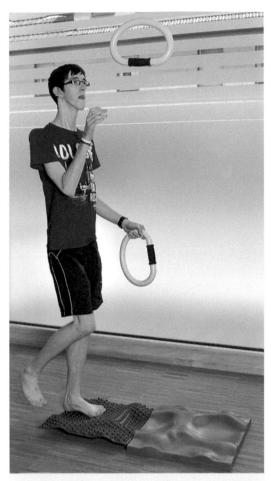

Fig. 6.66 Juggling on Terrasensa tiles.

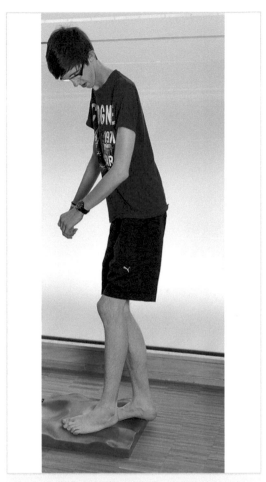

Fig. 6.67 Walking backward on Terrasensa tiles.

6.4.8 Sensamove

The Sensamove company offers various products for balance training. With the appropriate software, the degree of difficulty of training can be progressively increased. Patients can train in either a sitting or standing position. The motion sensors for the software and the software itself are compatible with equipment from other manufacturers, for example, with those supplied by Holz–Hörz.

6.5 Vibration Training

Jean-Marie Charcot (1825–1893), the French physiologist, described the therapeutic effect of vibrations on humans as early as the 19th century. He observed that the symptoms of patients with Parkinson's disease improved after a carriage ride on what back then were not very smooth roads.

The effect of vibrations on motor strength is the subject of some controversy in published studies. Some studies report a maximum increase in strength of up to 50% within 3 weeks, whereas others demonstrate an absent or only a slight increase in strength in similar training situations.[155]

Vibration training is also referred to as whole body vibration (WBV). The body's reaction to this motion depends on several different variables. The movement of the vibration plate plays an important role, as does the amplitude of plate motion. The third factor is the frequency that together with the amplitude acts on the body as an acceleration force. In our opinion, the frequency represents the decisive factor for the effect of training. The training should last no longer than 3 minutes, followed by a pause of 1 minute, and there should be three repetitions.

A vibrator unit should always be used within the scope of dual-task or multi-task training. This means

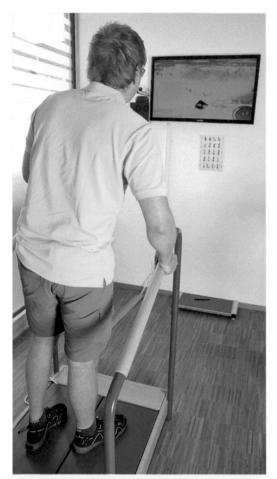

Fig. 6.68 MTD (measurement, therapy, documentation).

that the patient does not just stand on the vibrator unit but should also perform some other activity, such as turning the head, closing the eyes, shifting weight from one leg to the other, jumping from one leg to the other (well-rehabilitated patients), standing on one leg, or juggling.

Note

Fever disorders are an absolute contraindication for WBV. Relative contraindications for whole body vibration range from thrombosis, immediate postoperative phase, recent implants or fractures, acute inflammation, acute tendinopathy, acute hernia, acute discopathy, acute wounds or scars, active osteoarthritis and arthopathy, pregnancy, acute migraine, rheumatoid arthritis, epilepsy, and stone disorders of the biliary and urinary tracts to malignancies.[257]

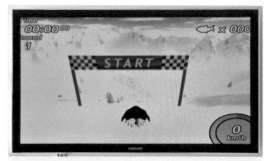

Fig. 6.69 MTD monitor.

Burkhardt[47] listed the effects of different frequencies in a table in an article. However, he only included units with a seesaw or vertical system (►Table 6.2). Ritzmann et al[342] showed that vibration alternating from one side to the other produced more pronounced activation of the electromyography leads than the synchronous vibration. However, Van Nes et al[415] published a study that failed to demonstrate any benefit from WBV with respect to balance and activities of daily life in comparison to the control group (training 5 days a week over a period of 6 weeks, 4 intervals of 45 seconds each on a Galileo 900, 3 mm amplitude and a frequency of 30 Hz).

6.5.1 SRT/Zeptor

Stochastic resonance therapy (SRT), formerly known as Zeptor, was developed at the Institute of Sports Science at the University of Frankfurt by Schmidbleicher and Haas. In stochastic resonance therapy, two plates vibrate independently and randomly in three dimensions. The frequency begins at 1 Hz and can be increased in increments of 0.1 Hz. Schmidtbleicher and Haas demonstrated the effectiveness of the Zeptor in different groups of patients in various publications. In 2002, they published a study that demonstrated an immediate effect of vibration training with the Zepter med in patients with Parkinson's disease. Following an intervention with vibration at an amplitude of 4 mm and a frequency of 4 to 6 Hz (5 applications of 1 minute each), they observed not only an improvement in various gait parameters but also in fine motor coordination tests. The effect persisted from 2 to 48 hours. In 20% of the patients, no effects were observed.[156] Additional positive effects were postulated for patients with Parkinson's disease using the Zeptoring.[407]

6.5.2 Galileo and Wellengang

Galileo, a seesaw vibration system, consists of a plate whose sides alternately move up and down. The new generation of Galileo machines begins at a frequency of 5 Hz. The vibration is continuous, and the amplitude can be varied by placing the patient's feet closer to or farther from the center.

Wellengang has further developed the seesaw technology. A spring suspension system flexibly supports the training platform at the central axis, adding a lateral excursion to the seesaw motion. The frequency can be reduced to 1 Hz and a slight stochastic deviation can be enabled as well. This makes it harder for the nervous system to become accustomed to the vibration.

6.5.3 Power Plate

Power Plate is a vibration plate that uses synchronous vibration; the vibration consists of an up-and-down motion with a frequency between 25 and 50 Hz. No scientific studies demonstrating an effect on patients with neurologic deficits are available, not even on the home page of Power Plate.

6.6 Climbing

Climbing, like walking, is a basal motion pattern. The training stress can be continuously adapted to the patient's individual level of performance. This flexible adaptation to motor ability and the low height of the climbing wall effectively eliminate the risk of injury or at least reduce it dramatically.

Therapeutic climbing is a form of therapy for improving physical deficits. Balance, agility, coordination, and strength are improved. Concentration and perception, creativity, and self-confidence are also increased. The patients climb on a wall as high as the room. Therapeutic climbing trains only

Table 6.2 Comparison of the effects of the Galileo system and the vertical system

Frequency	Galileo system	Vertical system
5–8 Hz	**Improvement of balance and proprioception**[46]	Not possible
10–15 Hz	**Improvement of perfusion**[204] Decrease in muscle tone Mobilization of joints Release of adhesions and scar tissue More rapid wound healing	Not possible
15–20 Hz	**Improvement of muscle strength**[29,46,264,377] **Improvement of coordination**[29,46,341] Improvement of stress incontinence[422] Improvement of constipation	Not possible
20–30 Hz	**Increase in bone density**[60,340] **Improvement of muscle strength**[29,40,209] **Improvement of coordination**[29] **Improvement in perfusion**[114] **Hormonal changes**[41] **Improvement of balance**[40,209] **Reduction of chronic lumbar back pain**[204] Increase in muscle tone Improvement in mobility Neurologic stimulation	(Only possible with certain models) **Improvement of muscle strength**[41,53] Hormonal changes[40] Increase in muscle tone Improvement of perfusion Improvement in mobility Neurologic stimulation
>30 Hz	Use of frequencies over 30 Hz on request. Note that the manufacturer does not recommend this	**Increase in bone density and improvement of muscle strength**[79] Increase in muscle tone Improvement of perfusion Improvement in mobility Neurologic stimulation

Note: Effects demonstrated in studies are shown in bold. Additional effects mentioned by the manufacturers appear in regular typeface.

Source: Burkhardt A. Vibrationstraining in der Physiotherapie–Wippen mit Wirkung. Physiopraxis 2006;9:22–24.

partial sequences from sports climbing. However, neurologic patients can also climb on a climbing wall in a sports center.

Kern demonstrated in a study that therapeutic climbing exerts positive effects on patients with multiple sclerosis.[203] Velikonja et al demonstrated in a study that sports climbing improves fatigue in patients with multiple sclerosis but has no effect on spasticity.[418] Lazik[229] published an article in which he demonstrated positive effects of therapeutic climbing on motor function in stroke patients after 12 therapy sessions in 6 weeks.

6.6.1 Climbing Wall (Boulder Wall)

A climbing wall is a helpful and financially justifiable investment for every physical therapy practice or rehabilitation facility. A climbing wall can be used with almost all patients, even with severely impaired neurologic patients. The climbing wall is an ideal piece of equipment for training leg strength in neurologic patients. The quadriceps can be very effectively strengthened in short sequences of functional training. With the external focus of tactile contact with the climbing wall, the patient automatically maintains the legs in external rotation.

Wall bars cannot replace the climbing wall. Wall bars differ from a climbing wall in that there exists a risk that the patient may slip off a rung. Nor can the leg assume the proper functional position on wall bars. Training on a climbing wall allows the patient to draw upon familiar motion patterns and to perform functional training of the whole body.

6.7 Small Devices for Training with Neurologic Patients

Many small devices can also be employed in therapeutic exercise in neurologic rehabilitation.

6.8 Slacklining

Slacklining (balancing on a slackline) was invented in Yosemite National Park, United States in the 1980s by the climbers, Adam Grosowsky and Jeff Ellington. Slacklining is the act of balancing on a suspended length of flat webbing about 3 cm wide. Initial attempts usually led to uncontrolled vibration of the weight-bearing leg. Slacklining has become very popular, and it is common to see young people in parks walking back and forth on unstable lengths of webbing. Many top athletes now train concentration, coordination, stability, and balance on a slackline.

Medicine has also discovered this sport. A few therapists and clinics use the slackline as a therapy device for treating certain disorders. Patients of every age suffering from craniocerebral trauma, stroke, multiple sclerosis, or Parkinson's disease can benefit from this form of therapy.

A decisive factor for therapy is the initial tension applied to the slackline that determines the amplitude and frequency with which the line moves under a dynamic load. Another essential factor is the length of the line. With a short slackline (less than 5 m), the amplitude remains small; the longer the slackline, the greater the amplitude, especially in the middle of the line. The length and tension of the slackline are the variables that can be changed according to the goal of therapy. If the focus of therapy is on leg strength, one should select a short, taut slackline. If the focus is on balance, one should opt for a longer one with less tension.

The therapy of neurologic patients begins with placing only one leg on the slackline followed by a gradual shift of more weight on this leg without causing the slackline to move. With two parallel slacklines, patients can also train in a quadruped stance. Additionally, the slackline offers patients an exciting and novel task involving fun that acts as a potentially motivating factor for them.

6.9 SilverFit

SilverFit is an exercise device for virtual rehabilitation. Many fitness exercises for training gross motor skills have been transformed into computer games so that patients have increased motivation to perform high number of repetitions. The unit is equipped with a three-dimensional (3D) camera that records the movements of up to four patients. This means that SilverFit doesn't require either a controller, mouse, or keyboard for training. The therapist can adapt the degree of difficulty of the exercises to the patient's respective performance level to ensure optimal training.

7 Clinical Pictures

7.1 Introduction

In this chapter, we present a few important clinical pictures in neurology. Along with a brief description of the pathophysiology and some general information, we present the respective symptoms and the measures that should be taken in therapeutic exercise. In addition to the most common clinical pictures, we also discuss a few less common ones with peculiarities that require special consideration in therapeutic exercise regimes. This list of clinical pictures is by no means comprehensive. However, by considering the individual symptoms, the reader should be able to draw conclusions about how other clinical pictures not discussed in this chapter should be dealt with in therapeutic exercise and realize which precautions must be taken.

7.2 Stroke

Definition []

The World Health Organization (WHO, 1989) defines stroke as "rapidly developing clinical signs of focal (or global) disturbance of cerebral function, with symptoms lasting 24 hours or longer or leading to death, with no apparent cause other than vascular origin."

Stroke is the third most common cause of death in industrialized countries. The incidence of stroke in Germany, and possibly globally, is approximately 200 per 100,000 individuals. An acute focal neurologic deficit due to a circumscribed interruption of the blood supply to the brain is referred to as an ischemic stroke. The term "cerebrovascular insult" is used synonymously; the term "apoplexy" is obsolete. The term "cerebral infarct" describes the morphologic correlation of cerebral parenchymal necrosis, which with today's imaging modalities can be demonstrated in living patients.[86]

Seventy-five percent of all stroke patients also suffer from a cardiovascular disorder.[346] The question of whether therapeutic exercise and sports are recommended in rehabilitation has since long been answered for patients with coronary heart disease, such as those who have suffered a myocardial infarction or undergone bypass surgery.[261] Although the risk factors and pathophysiologic processes are similar for poststroke patients and patients with coronary artery disease, the approaches in rehabilitation are entirely different. The focus of rehabilitation of patients with cardiovascular disease is on physical training. These patients know that they must regain strength, endurance, and fitness.[261] The stroke patients are no longer able to perform certain activities of daily life that require greater expenditure of energy. This is due in part to physical inactivity.[196,259] The improvement in care in the acute phase (in stroke units) has decreased mortality in the 10 years from 1998 to 2008 by about 40% from 150 to 90 per 100,000.[339] The effect of this has been that the number of people with many persistent motor deficits has continuously increased in the recent years.

The maximum oxygen intake of stroke patients is significantly reduced in comparison with inactive control persons of the same age.[330] Although it is known that stroke patients can significantly improve their cardiovascular load tolerance with aerobic training, many physical therapy and occupational therapy concepts have yet to put this knowledge into practice.[262,146]

The extent and severity of the disability depend on the location and distribution of the damage. Additional prognostic indicators also allow prediction of the extent of functional recovery. As early as 1986, Granger et al[151] demonstrated the value of urinary and fecal incontinence as a prognostic indicator. Every subsequent study has shown urinary incontinence persisting beyond day 7 to be an unfavorable prognostic indicator for both mortality and independence after 3 months.[118] The frequent use of indwelling urinary catheters in stroke units has largely eliminated the relevance of this prognostic indicator. The presence of difficulties in swallowing is also an important prognostic indicator for mortality and morbidity. However, this factor has only been examined in a few studies. The 50 mL water test has become an established method for verifying difficulties in swallowing. This involves successive swallowing of 5 mL of water with and without pulse oximetry and watching for voice changes, coughing, or choking fits.

The evaluation of motor skills (strength, endurance, control of movement) was also examined in several studies; especially the strength for making a fist has proven to be a good prognostic indicator for the ability to grasp objects. The increase in strength in the paretic leg muscles and the increasing control over simple or complex voluntary movements, especially those near the trunk, are leading indicators of the subsequent ability to walk with or without aids.[118]

Many patients have motor deficits after a stroke and are thus restricted in their mobility. The "traditional" physical therapy treatment concepts based on neurophysiology are centered on the treatment of one factor of the upper motor neuron syndrome. These therapeutic options focus on normalizing the muscle tone (reducing spasticity).

The pathophysiologic cause of patients' motor problems after a stroke is the damage to the upper motor neuron. Jackson[197] divided the complex symptoms of an upper motor neuron lesion into plus and minus symptoms (▶Fig. 7.1) that can occur concomitantly or successively in varying severity. The minus symptoms usually occur immediately after the event, whereas the plus symptoms tend to develop only over the course of time. The minus symptoms cause significant functional deficits.

Although there are many hypotheses about spasticity, its cause has yet to be completely explained. Diener and Putzki[89] demonstrated that an intrinsic change in the muscle fibers occurs in spastic muscles. O'Dwyer et al[284] demonstrated as early as 1996 that spasticity as defined by Lance rarely occurs after stroke, but almost all patients have shortening of the muscles.[6]

An increasing number of studies note the importance of minus symptoms for motor activity. Based on sequential measurements of the strength of making a fist, a study by Sunderlad et al[386] demonstrated that strength is a good indicator for predicting improvement of function in situations of daily life. The strength of the hip flexors and plantar flexors directly influences the walking speed and poststroke patients have decreased maximum strength and slower power generation in the elbow flexors and extensors on the affected side.[279,51]

The question of whether specific strength training is helpful to poststroke patients has been answered positively by many studies.[268,393,400] Recent studies, too, have shown that specific strength training can lead to improvements in mobility and activities of daily life.[234,124,11] Flansbjer et al[123] demonstrated the effect of progressive resistance training in poststroke patients in a 4-year follow-up study.

The preferred pattern of motion in patients with hemiplegia can be observed as an optimal adaptation of the motor system to the given situation rather than as a "pathologic" behavior.[226] If we accept that the pattern of motion in stroke patients is the optimal adaptation to their motor capabilities

---

Definition   []

Lance[224] explains spasticity as: "Spasticity is a motor disorder with increased velocity-dependent resistance to passive motion."

Upper motor neuron syndrome

• Plus symptoms	• Minus symptoms
• Spasticity	• Paresis, weakness, paralysis
• Clonus	• Fine motor dysfunction
• Increased reflexes	• Dysdiadochokinesia, slowness
• Babinski's sign	• Increased effort, rapid exhaustion
• Associated reactions	• Limited automatic movements
• Mass movements	• Difficulty in dual tasks

Spasticity is almost invariably associated with paresis of variable severity.

Fig. 7.1 Upper motor neuron syndrome: plus and minus symptoms.

after a stroke, we must also accept that a stroke patient does not have the option of walking in any different way. Improving performance in walking will only be possible if the patient trains walking, receives the necessary aids, and can then draw on a better pattern of motion. We only learn to walk by practicing it.

7.2.1 What Training Should a Stroke Patient Perform?

A large percentage of stroke patients have cardiovascular problems, and almost all chronic stroke patients exhibit deconditioning syndrome. As movements are difficult for them to perform, these patients tend to move less and exhibit learned nonuse.

The primary goal of poststroke patients is almost always to improve their mobility. As rehabilitation progresses, the focus is expanded to include dexterity in the upper extremities and further improvement of gait components as training and therapy goals only. Even poststroke patients can reach a point during rehabilitation where they want to resume participating in sports activities at a high level of performance. Thus, training should include all basic motor skills, always in a manner appropriate to the patient's level of performance.

Patients in the early phase are able to perform treadmill training with a body weight–supported system (BWST). This treadmill training is either output controlled and measured in watts or pulse controlled, depending on what the attending physician prescribes. As soon as possible, the patient should be encouraged not to hold on to the railing so that training increasingly involves unassisted walking. Walking training should be performed in dual-task or multi-task mode at an early stage. The patient also trains carrying objects, turning the head, simultaneously speaking, or performing other cognitive tasks. Endurance training can also be performed on a recumbent ergometer. Strength training on a leg press or a climbing wall should be included. The stroke patient must be able to move at least his or her own body weight both concentrically and eccentrically several times in a coordinated manner.

> **Note**
>
> In general, we may say that the following muscle groups are particularly weak in stroke patients:
> - Quadriceps
> - Calf
> - Lateral trunk
> - Muscles of the proximal shoulder girdle

How can we conclude that these muscles, in particular, are weak in a stroke patient? Many stroke patients can be observed to hyperextend the knee when walking or standing. This hyperextension is necessary for these patients because they lack the strength to perform an effective knee extension for a longer period of time. Since calf muscles constitute a group of muscles responsible for quick walking, their weakness prevents the patients from walking at a high speed. Weakness in the trunk muscles is apparent from asymmetry when standing or even sitting without support. Several patients exhibit good distal function in the upper extremity but lack a proximal integration of the arm. Therefore, training with an upper body ergometer or other strength components should be included for the upper extremities. One may attempt to manage a painful shoulder with tape or by changing the radius to achieve pain-free movement. A study by Neupert and Hamzei[281] demonstrated the efficacy of taping with kinesio tape for shoulder pain in poststroke patients.

Many stroke patients have such severe paresis in the arm that they are unable to train on their own. Robot-assisted training is necessary in these cases, as there is limited time for a one-on-one situation (one therapist to one patient). An additional advantage of robot-assisted training is that motion behavior and motor recovery can be automatically measured.[421]

> **Note**
>
> The following goals can also be achieved or expected in therapeutic exercise regimes for rehabilitating poststroke patients[262]:
> - Increasing activity and preventing complications from inactivity.
> - Decreasing the risk of recurrent stroke and cardiac events.
> - Increasing cardiovascular fitness.
> - Improving muscle strength.

These considerations show that training and sports activities should increasingly be recommended in the future as a part of poststroke neurorehabilitation. In Germany, training guidelines exist for patients with cardiovascular deficits but the national guidelines for poststroke rehabilitation do not contain any explicit references to cardiovascular training. In the United States, the American College of Sports Medicine Physical Activity (ACSMPA) and the American Heart Association (AHA) defined goals and exercise intensity levels for aerobic training in their guidelines for stroke patients back in 2004.[262]

The following points should be considered when recruiting poststroke patients for aerobic training[263]:

- Patients should undergo a cardiologic examination and an exercise test prior to endurance training.
- Patients should take their medications before beginning training and refrain from eating for 2 hours before the beginning of training.
- Training should take place at an appropriate time of day such as in the morning. A training record should be kept.
- Training should occur 3 to 5 times a week and should last for at least 30 minutes including warm up and cool down.
- Training intensity should be 50 to 80% of the maximum heart rate.
- Results of tests such as the 6 minute or the 10 meter walking test should be documented.
- It may be important for patients to change their lifestyle to ensure long-term maintainance of results.

In a meta-analysis in 2006, Pang et al found that fitness training after a stroke resulted in the following improvements[293]:

- Improvement in the maximum oxygen consumption improved.
- Increased maximum walking speed increased.
- Coverage of a longer distance in the 6 minute walking test.

Sauders et al demonstrated in a meta-analysis that cardiorespiratory training significantly increased the walking speed and walking endurance and reduced dependence on walking aids.[350]

Walking training should be performed 3 to 5 days a week for 20 to 40 minutes at 50 to 80% of heart rate reserve.[146] Even patients in the chronic stage benefit from training. This holds true even if the patient only begins 3 to 12 months after the insult, albeit to a lesser extent.[96,380]

Equipment can be used even in the early phase to begin early mobilization and rehabilitation of stroke patients. Bedridden patients can train both arms and legs passively, with assistance, and actively with the MOTOmed letto 2 (▶Fig. 7.2). The GIGER MD can also be utilized for effective therapy in the early phase as well as in the later phase of rehabilitation (▶Fig. 7.3). The Erigo by Hocoma is a good device for mobilizing patients out of bed in the early phase. In the Erigo, the patient is brought into an upright position while his or her legs are in passive motion, and dynamic loading and relaxation cycles are applied. This means that the patient experiences an intensive training session even in the early phase of rehabilitation (▶Fig. 7.4).

Even in the early phase, the focus of rehabilitation is on improving walking ability. The stroke patient must regain the postural control. Postural control can only be trained when the patient has to deal with gravity. Standing places demands higher postural control and balance than walking because walking is a basal motion pattern. For the

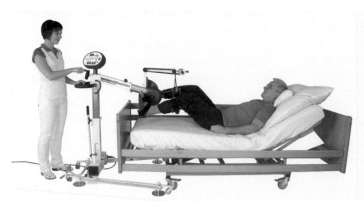

Fig. 7.2 MOTOmed Letto 2. Used with the kind permission of RECK-Technik GmbH & Co. KG, Betzenweiler, Germany.

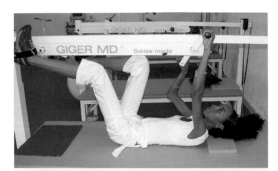

Fig. 7.3 Giger MD. Used with the kind permission of Combo AG, Tugginerweg 3, Solothurn, Switzerland, www.gigermd.com.

rehabilitation of stroke patients, this means that they should walk as soon as possible, even with body weight–supporting systems on the treadmill or with the Lokomat. Two aspects are important in improving walking ability, speed and endurance. Speed can be improved considerably with interval training.[319]

7.2.2 Why Strength Training in Poststroke Rehabilitation?

Prado–Medeiros et al[321] found significant strength deficits in the knee extensors and flexors in post-stroke patients, implying that even stroke patients needed specific strength training. Like all neurologic patients, stroke patients have strength deficits. In stroke patients, the deficits usually involve the following muscles:

- Dorsiflexors
- Calf muscles
- Knee extensors
- Lateral trunk muscles
- Scapular muscles
- Elbow flexors and extensors
- Finger flexors and extensors

Therefore, it is important in stroke patients to perform Medical Research Council (MRC) tests of muscular function according to the patient's goals. In the MRC test, one should test from reflex inhibiting positions. The test is also performed as an isometric task to prevent the patient from exploiting movements of mass.

Stroke patients can utilize all the strength training equipment that healthy persons employ. However, the equipment must allow adjustments to be

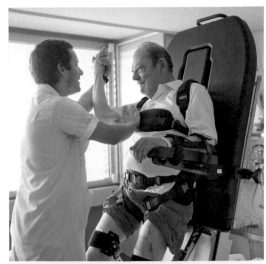

Fig. 7.4 Erigo. Used with the kind permission of Hocoma, Volketswil, Switzerland.

made. Stroke patients can improve the strength of the leg extensors with the leg press; single-leg training is also important. Treadmill training with an uphill incline set is a good way to train the muscles of the calves. Walking sideways on a treadmill strengthens both the abductors of the lower leg and trains eversion of the upper foot more effectively. The climbing wall is good for training the knee extensors in a functional initial position. An upper body ergometer or cycling trainer can be used for training the upper extremity. The shoulder muscles are exercised with a butterfly reverse unit, a rowing machine, or on the climbing wall. The trunk muscles can be trained with a feedback-controlled trunk trainer, on a rowing machine with a boom, or in a functional setting, on the climbing wall. Strengthening the trunk muscles results in a better postural control, which in turn, improves walking (▶ Fig. 7.5).

7.2.3 Why Endurance Training in Rehabilitation of Stroke Patients?

As was discussed above, the majority of stroke patients suffer from cardiovascular problems. As the requirements for mobility after a stroke are higher than before it, stroke patients require better strength and muscular endurance than healthy persons of the same age. The strength required increases as the walking speed decreases.

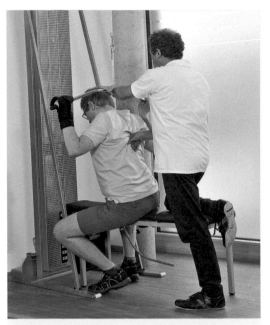

Fig. 7.5 Trunk training with a Lat-pull machine.

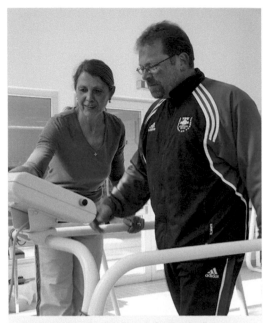

Fig. 7.6 Endurance training on the treadmill.

Movements are more strenuous when the patient need to overcome the resistance of hypertonic musculature. Specific endurance training may be performed on ergometers, treadmills, or during activities of daily life such as climbing stairs. All types of training help to improve participation in social activities (▶Fig. 7.6).

7.3 Multiple Sclerosis

<table>
<tr><td>Definition</td><td>[ ]</td></tr>
<tr><td colspan="2">Multiple sclerosis is a chronic inflammatory neuro-degenerative disease characterized by demyelin-ation of the nerves in the brain and spinal cord.</td></tr>
</table>

The prevalence of multiple sclerosis in Germany is about 120 per 100,000 individuals.[81] The most important motor impairments in multiple sclerosis include pareses, spasticity, and ataxia.[223] Of these, the pareses are most prominent, both at the onset of the disease and during its subsequent course.[20] Spasticity is not an early sign of multiple sclerosis; however, in the further course of the disorder spasticity has been reported to occur in 60 to 70% of all patients.[169]

The recent literature frequently refers to the upper motor neuron syndrome (UMNS). Pareses, reduced muscular endurance, slowed movements, and reduced fine motor control are referred to as minus symptoms; heightened intrinsic reflexes, increased muscle tone, pyramidal tract signs, clonus, and associated reflexes are referred to as plus symptoms.[197] We must assume that spasticity and paresis are different syndromes of UMNS; however, it has been shown that both symptoms occur together and influence each other. Paresis is far more problematic for all patients than spasticity because it is far more difficult or maybe even impossible to perform a transfer with paresis than with spasticity.

There is a certain order in which paresis affects the muscles. At the onset of the disorder, weakness is detectable in the dorsiflexors in the ankle, followed by the hip flexors and the muscles of the lower anterior abdomen.[223] Therefore, these muscles must be trained for strength and muscular endurance.

Patients can use the following method to train dorsiflexion of the foot themselves: The patient stands with his or her back close to the wall and with the trunk extended leans backward. As soon as the patient's body passes behind the coronal plane, the dorsiflexors reactively respond to prevent a backward fall. Even when leaning against the wall, the patient can train the dorsiflexors by shifting his or her weight back onto the feet. It is important to initiate the movement from the pelvis. Another good exercise for foot dorsiflexion is to tap the foot in time to music.[223] Climbing stairs is a good way to train the hip flexors.

Another important symptom of multiple sclerosis is fatigue. Many MS patients say that this tiredness is the most annoying symptom for activities of daily life. Various different pathogenetic mechanisms have been suggested to explain this feeling of exhaustion in MS patients. Immunologic factors have also been suspected as the cause (cytokines have been detected). Deconditioning syndrome as a result of reduced activity could also play a role.[418]

As walking ability is an important indicator for a favorable clinical course of the disorder, therapeutic exercise can cover one crucial point required for a favorable clinical course. Studies of patients with MS report that treadmill training can achieve positive effects.[223] Patients with MS should refrain from stretching or warming up prior to treadmill training, as the patient may have too little muscle tone and therefore unable to walk. Walking is also crucial for the trunk muscles, as every step represents functional training for these muscles. Patients in wheelchairs should especially and regularly perform treadmill training. Retaining walking ability is a favorable prognostic indicator against progression of the disorder.

Patients with MS should complete treadmill training to improve their endurance and walking speed. Patients should walk at what they feel is an optimal speed until they tire, followed by taking a short break (about 1–2 minutes) and repeating the whole sequence two more times. The important thing for the patients is to keep the Borg scale in mind so that they train optimally irrespective of their daily ups and downs.

The treadmill should be set at an incline for patients with MS, thereby allowing them to better compensate for the weakness of their foot dorsiflexors. Patients with MS can also benefit from a foot orthosis if they have difficulty advancing the foot due to weakness in the dorsiflexors. However, this orthosis may have only minimal weight. As soon as patients with MS no longer walk regularly, weakening of the trunk musculature occurs as a result of learned nonuse. For this reason, all patients with MS who primarily rely on a wheelchair to get around should take part in regular walking training, in necessary with a body weight–support system.

Therapy must take this into consideration the fact that some patients with MS also suffer from the Uhthoff phenomenon. The Uhthoff phenomenon is the exacerbation of existing symptoms or the appearance of new symptoms with a rise in body temperature. These symptoms resolve as soon as body temperature has returned to normal. The phenomenon is the reason that patients with MS are advised to avoid strenuous activities. However, patients suffering from the Uhthoff phenomenon can and should exercise. Patients can exercise with cooling vests and must be made to understand that the Uhthoff phenomenon is a reversible impairment.

Note

There is no evidence whatsoever that training or even physical overexertion might trigger an acute episode in patients with MS.

Well planned pauses are decisively important in exercise regimes for patients with MS suffering from fatigue. A brief pause of about 1–2 minutes will suffice for most patients. Many studies demonstrate that aerobic training has a positive effect on fatigue.[302,87,274,344] Studies of sports activities also demonstrate a positive effect on fatigue.[286,143] Motl et al[275] showed that patients with MS who were physically more active suffered less from depression and fatigue and had a better social environment and greater self-confidence. The last few years have witnessed a sharp increase in the number of studies of strength and/or endurance training with patients with MS.

Patients with MS who exercised on a treadmill three times a week over a period of 4 weeks were able to significantly improve both their walking speed and walking endurance. This was not accompanied by any worsening of fatigue.[413] Walking speed is particularly dependent on the strength of the calf musculature, as these muscle groups provide the power to move the leg forward.

The following recommendations can be deduced from various studies of the effect of strength training on patients with MS:

- Training should be conducted at least two or three times a week. When the patients are in a better shape, training frequency should be increased to four times a week.
- A training session should last 10–40 minutes.
- It is a good idea to alternate between strength training and endurance training.[73,302,343,362]

To date, no study has shown any connection, neither a significant one nor even a trend, between physical activity and the occurrence of an acute episode.[303]

Practical Tip

General Principles for Training with Multiple Sclerosis Patients:

- An optimal training interval is 3 to 4 times a week but at least twice a week.
- Training time per session should be at least 20–30 minutes. Total training time per week should not be less than 60 minutes.[184,423]
- With regard to training intensity, patients should follow the Borg scale and train for about 10–15 minutes (►Fig. 7.7).
- In addition to the number of repetitions and the weights used, the pause duration is an important factor in training patients with MS. The pause duration depends on the size of the muscles trained and the complexity and degree of difficulty of the task. The pause duration should be between half the training time (for simple motion sequences or small muscle groups) and twice the training time (for complex patterns of motion or large muscle groups).[223]

In each training session, the patient should train endurance, strength, and coordination. The emphasis varies according to the distribution of symptoms, the patient's shape on that day, and the manner of performance. Stretching should be incorporated into the training sequence as required.

6	
7	Very, very light
8	
9	Very light
10	
11	Fairly light
12	
13	Somewhat hard
14	
15	Hard
16	
17	Very hard
18	
19	Very, very hard
20	

Fig. 7.7 Borg scale for evaluating subjective fatigue.

Practical Tip

Principles for Effective Strength Training with Multiple Sclerosis Patients[223]:

- Little weight, many repetitions.
- Include functional leg training, for example, on the treadmill or climbing wall.
- Pay attention to the leg axis.
- Include pauses (fatigue).
- Pay attention to compensatory movement patterns.
- Pay attention to reflex-inhibiting initial positions and body temperature (cooling vests).
- First increase the number of repetitions, then the weights.

Mulcare recommends adapting the training plan for patients with MS every 6 months.[276]

Dalgas[73] based on his review, gives the following training recommendations to patients with MS with an Expanded Disability Status Scale (EDSS) value greater than 7:

- Patients with MS should consult a physical therapist before beginning a new training program.
- The program must be individually structured.
- Strength training should be performed under supervision until the patient is familiar with the training program.
- Closed chain exercises should be used initially.
- Fifteen repetitions should be possible at the beginning of training.
- The intensity should be such that a maximum of 8–15 repetitions can be performed. After a few months, intensity should be increased so that 8–10 repetitions are possible.
- The number of sets should initially be 1–3 per exercise.
- After a few months, the number of sets should be increased to 3–4 per exercise.
- The pauses between the sets should be 2–4 minutes.
- The training program should include 4–8 exercises.
- The frequency of training should be 2 to 3 times a week.
- Large muscle groups should be trained first followed by small ones. Exercises involving several joints are performed first followed by exercises involving a single joint.

- Training the lower extremities takes priority over training the upper extremities.
- Strength training should alternate with endurance training.

The focus of training changes with severely impaired patients. Patients who are unable to walk must stand for at least 1 hour each day for effective prophylaxis. Additionally, trunk training and strength in the upper extremities including the shoulder musculature becomes more important. Strength in the upper extremities has a decisive impact on the independence of patients confined to a wheelchair. These patients are able to perform a transfer on their own only in the presence of sufficient strength in their upper body and arms.

However, this does not mean that patients severely affected with MS should not train their legs. Training the legs with a cycling trainer can have a good effect on spasticity. Training with a cycling trainer should always include exercising against resistance.

Filipi et al[119] demonstrated that patients with MS benefit from strength training regardless of the severity of the disorder. For the study, they divided the patients into three groups:
- Group 1: Patients with an EDSS score of 1.0 to 4.5.
- Group 2: Patients with an EDSS score of 5.0–7.0.
- Group 3: Patients with an EDSS score greater than 7.5.

The patients were trained in 50-minute sessions twice a week for 6 months. Training took place in groups and one therapist supervised three persons. Following a warm-up phase of about 5 to 10 minutes, the patients completed an approximately 30-minute individual interval training program focusing on strength, power generation, and balance. The intensity of the exercises was chosen to allow the candidates to complete two to three sets with 10 repetitions. This was followed by a cooldown period involving static stretching of the various muscle groups for about 5 to 10 minutes. After 6 months of training, all the patients, regardless of the severity of their disorder according to their EDSS score, exhibited a significant improvement in all the strength parameters.

7.4 Parkinson's Disease

The prevalence of Parkinson's disease can be assumed to be approximately 100 to 200 per 100,000 individuals. However, the prevalence varies greatly with age. The prevalence in Germany among persons aged between 70 and 74 is about 700 per 100,000 individuals, whereas among those aged between 75 and 79, it is about 1,800 per 100,000 individuals.[85] Only about 4% of patients are younger than 50 years at the onset of the disorder. After the 50th year of life, the risk of developing Parkinson's disease increases each year by 9%, meaning that a 60-year-old person has a 90% higher risk of developing Parkinson's disease than a 50-year-old.

> **Note**
>
> Parkinson's disease is characterized by a combination of motor and nonmotor symptoms. The main motor symptoms are often more pronounced on one side (hemi-Parkinson) and include[105]:
> - Bradykinesia
> - Rigor
> - Resting tremor
> - Postural instability

In spite of improvement and further development in pharmaceutical treatments and brain-stimulation therapy, the majority of patients with Parkinson's disease develops severe disabilities in the course of the disorder. Activating therapies, such as physical therapy and occupational therapy management of swallowing, and logopedics become increasingly important as the disorder progresses because pharmacologic treatments can only insufficiently influence balance, walking, speaking, swallowing, and cognitive problems over the long term.[56]

The fundamental problem of motor impairments in patients with Parkinson's disease is the impaired execution of automatic movement patterns.[105] This means that the focus in motor rehabilitation of patients with Parkinson's disease must be on the impaired automation and rhythm of motion sequences, the reduced speed and amplitude of the individual movements, and the derangement of posture and postural stability.

Patients with Parkinson's disease have less muscular strength than the healthy persons of the same age.[214,282,52] Even in the early stages of the disorder (transition from stage I to stage II according to Hoehn and Yahr,[181] ▶Table 7.1), patients tend to give up sports activities and strenuous physical tasks such as working in the garden.[333] These findings help to define the goals of training with patients with Parkinson's disease.

Table 7.1 Hoehn–Yahr scale

Stages	Severity of the disorder
Stage 0	No signs of disease
Stage 1	Unilateral disease
Stage 1.5	Unilateral disease and involvement of the axis of the body
Stage 2	Bilateral disease without balance impairment
Stage 2.5	Slight bilateral disease without compensation during pull test
Stage 3	Slight to moderate bilateral disease. There is slight postural instability but the patient is still physically independent
Stage 4	Severe disability. The patient can still walk or stand without assistance
Stage 5	Without assistance, the patient is confined to the wheelchair or bed

An increasing number of studies show that patients with Parkinson's disease benefit from physical activity.[180,68,147,273,13] Treadmill training with and without body weight–support systems[270,170,260] and vibration training[157,103] can produce short-term improvements in gait and balance parameters. Treadmill therapy can also produce long-term effects that are relevant to daily life. Scandalis et al[351] demonstrated that strength training in the trunk and legs could improve gait. Strength and endurance training combined with stretching can prevent axial deformities. However, these effects can only be achieved with long-term training at frequent intervals.

Patients with Parkinson's disease have an increased risk of falling in dual-task situations.[316] Therefore, one should carefully consider which situations patients with Parkinson's disease should practice dual tasks in.[316] Therapeutic exercise regimes should train large, high-amplitude movements with a high number of repetitions (LSVT BIG)[116] One study showed that training with a cycling trainer at a speed of 90 rpm led to good improvements in motor status in patients with Parkinson's disease.[336] These cycling trainers are manufactured by Reck and distributed under the name MOTOmed viva 2 Parkinson.

Physical activity in patients with Parkinson's disease stimulates the increased secretion of dopamine, which, in turn, promotes neuroplasticity and the structural adaptation of nerve cells.[147,13]

Note

Treadmill therapy has also been shown to be superior to conventional physical therapy for patients with Parkinson's disease. [264,273]

The structured speed-dependent treadmill training (STT) described in Chapter 6.2.1 can improve walking speed and the length of stride even in patients with Parkinson's disease.[320]

Scandalis et al[351] demonstrated that consistent strength training of the trunk and legs led to an improvement in muscular strength, length of stride, walking speed, and posture. Patients with slight to moderately severe disease were able to achieve a level of strength similar to that of the healthy persons of the same age. Pendt et al[299] demonstrated that patients with Parkinson's disease training a throwing task are able to achieve accuracy and reliability comparable to control persons of the same age. However, the effect of practice did not persist for long among patients with Parkinson's disease as in the control group. Thus, patients with Parkinson's disease had to begin the next training session at a level lower than the control group.[299] This indicates that the best effects of training with patients with Parkinson's disease can be achieved with regular and frequent training.

Given the evidence that physical activity has both neuroplastic and protective effects on patients with Parkinson's disease, we may reasonably expect that in the future, persons with Parkinson's disease will receive activating therapies early in the course of the disorder and not when functionally relevant disabilities occur.[332]

The fundamental problem of motor impairments in patients with Parkinson's disease is the impaired execution of automatic movement patterns. The result is that set shifting, switching from one set of movements to another, is rendered difficult and is only performed very slowly. The repetitive performance or sequencing of movements is impaired, becoming reduced and irregular. Also, motor function can be positively and negatively influenced by external stimuli or cues.[105] This also defines the goals of therapeutic exercise regimes for patients with Parkinson's disease.

> **Note**
>
> The main focus of training should be on the following items:
> - Improving the impaired automation and rhythm of motion sequences.
> - Increasing the amplitude of motion and the speed of motion and walking.
> - Improving posture and postural stability.

The important thing about improving postural stability is that patients with Parkinson's disease need training in postural stability with shifting balance, that is, they need mobile stability. Two weeks of two daily 20-minute sessions of repetitive, selective training of protective steps significantly improved both the size of the protective step and the reaction time.[199] Hirsch et al[180] demonstrated that patients, who underwent regular combined training (alternating strength and balance training) achieved a greater improvement than patients who underwent balance training alone.

The goals of improving mobile stability, increasing the amplitude of motion, and increasing the speed of motion require both strength training and endurance training. Every training session should initiate with stretching the various muscle groups, which tend to be shortened due to the typical posture of patients with Parkinson's disease. This means that the anterior musculature of the trunk, leg muscles, and the shoulder and neck muscles must be stretched (▶Fig. 7.8). Patients with Parkinson's disease must be guided and convinced that they should also perform these exercises at home.

A strength training program for patients with Parkinson's disease primarily includes the knee extensors on the leg press, including single-leg exercises with at least patient's own body weight, and the trunk extensors with exercises on an unstable surface. However, the program also aims to increase the strength in the upper extremities. Rowing machines and butterfly reverse units are well suited for this purpose as are the cycling trainers. An axial deformity in patients with Parkinson's disease requires intensive and continuous

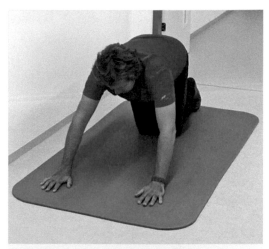

Fig. 7.8 Stretching for patients with Parkinson's disease on the hands and knees.

attention with the focus on strength training combined with appropriate stretching exercises.

LSVT BIG is a relatively new training and therapy method. Patients are instructed to perform large, high-amplitude, stereotypical motions with the therapist. Here again, highly repetitive training is necessary. These movements are combined with stretching exercises. With its intensive repetition and constant monitoring by the therapist, BIG enables patients to access untapped motion reserves and consciously apply them to daily life.

Patients perform at least 12 different whole-body BIG motions with at least 10 repetitions in every therapy session. Intensive repetition of the exercises and constant feedback about the results achieved activates and expands the patient's untapped capacities. The therapist motivates the patient to perform each motion with the greatest possible effort ("at least 80% of maximum energy") and with appreciable exertion.[104] Thus, patients with Parkinson's disease should train in the range of up to 17 on the Borg scale. Wherever possible, BIG training should be initiated in the early phase of idiopathic Parkinson's disease and should also be continued in an outpatient setting.

If possible, training should be conducted in the "on" phase. Patients should be instructed to keep a motion log, in which the on and off phases are recorded (▶Table 7.2).

Table 7.2 Motion log for patients with Parkinson's disease

Medications	Time	Ability to move on day						
		1	2	3	4	5	6	7
	06:00–07:00 am							
	07:00–08:00 am							
	08:00–09:00 am							
	09:00–10:00 am							
	10:00–11:00 am							
	11:00–12:00 am							
	12:00–1:00 pm							
	1:00–2:00 pm							
	2:00–3:00 pm							
	3:00–4:00 pm							
	4:00–5:00 pm							
	5:00–6:00 pm							
	6:00–7:00 pm							
	7:00–8:00 pm							
	8:00–9:00 pm							
	9:00–10:00 pm							
	10:00–11:00 pm							
	11:00–12:00 pm							
	Night							

+ = Good mobility; ○ = moderate mobility; - = poor mobility; × = hyperkinesis.

> **Note**
>
> External cues should be employed in training with patients with Parkinson's disease. Acoustic, visual, or tactile cues can and should be used, especially in treadmill therapy and with patients who experience gait "freezing" to increase walking speed and make the step sequence more rhythmical.[249]

Freezing greatly curtails self-reliance and is responsible for 25% of falls with serious consequences in patients with Parkinson's disease.[103] The therapist can and should "trigger" the beginning of the motion with visual, acoustic, and/or sensory stimuli and instruct the patient how to use these tricks in daily life as well. Gait training with acoustic or visual cues can also improve the stride length and walking speed both during training and afterward.[352] Ebersbach and Ceballos–Baumann[103] recommend the following areas of emphasis for training with patients with Parkinson's disease:

- Training with sensory cues.
- **Balance training:** This is usually combined with strength and endurance training so that it becomes difficult to demonstrate a clear effect of the balance training. Different initial positions should be utilized in balance training depending on the severity of the disorder. It is important to remember that patients with Parkinson's disease have greater problems with balance when they are cognitively distracted. It is crucial to take this into consideration while training. Balance training rates about 10 to 12 on the Borg scale in terms of subjective exertion. Training should also be conducted with the eyes closed or with head movements, and also in a walking position or on an unstable surface. The exercises should be varied and each should last about 20–30 seconds. The entire training session should be about 20 to 40 minutes with two to three sessions a week.

- **Strength and endurance training:** A combination of light endurance and strength training has proven to be optimal for patients with Parkinson's disease. Treadmill training at a low speed for a long period is more effective than training at a higher speed for a shorter period.[367] Endurance training should be conducted three to five times a week for about 20 to 40 times, not including warm up and cool down. Training intensity should be about 60 to 80% of the maximum heart rate. Walking speed on the treadmill at the beginning of training should be at least 60% of walking speed achieved in the 6-minute walking test, whereas subjective exertion can be about 11–13 on the Borg scale. Strength training should be conducted in combination with endurance training. Training should include 4 to 10 exercises, each in one to three series of 8 to 15 repetitions. Subjective exertion on the Borg scale can be about 15 to 17. If the patient exceeds the required number of repetitions, the weight should be increased. Strength training focuses on the lower extremities and the trunk. This means that particular attention should be paid to the triceps surae, quadriceps, gluteus maximus, and posterior trunk muscles. After specific training on equipment to strengthen these muscles, the patient can also be instructed to include appropriate exercises in a home training program (▶Fig. 7.9).
- **Cognitive motion strategies:** As patients with Parkinson's disease face difficulty with the automated execution of complex motions, such complex motions can be subdivided into individual elements by cognitive cues. These elements are then subdivided into defined sequences consisting of relatively simple motion elements. The result is that complex motions are split up in a manner to allow the activities to be performed consciously. Double tasks are avoided in these complex activities of daily life; the individual motions are practiced and memorized. The goal is not to automate the motion of activity, as it must be consciously controlled. Cues can make it easier to initiate the motion or activity. Standing up from a chair is one such example. The patient with Parkinson's disease does not simply stand up. The patient first shifts his or her weight to the right foot, then to the left, then back to the right, then back to the left, then counts "1, 2, 3," followed by standing up. Additional acoustic

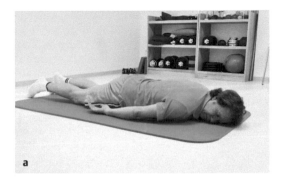

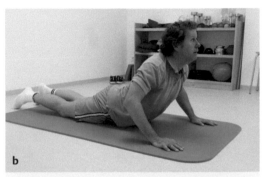

Fig. 7.9 Home exercises for patients with Parkinson's disease.

stimuli, such as clapping the hands or slapping the thigh, are added as needed.

7.5 Paraplegia

Paraplegia results from damage to the spinal cord and/or cauda equina. Motor, sensory, and vegetative deficits occur distal to the injury. Paraplegia is usually caused by an accident. The incidence of traumatic injuries in the industrialized countries is 10 to 30 per million (Guideline of the German Society of Neurology [in German]; 2012; paraplegia; AWMF register number: 030/070).

In 1944, Ludwig Guttmann (1899–1980) opened a treatment center for paraplegic patients in Stoke Mandeville, England, where he and his team developed the fundamentals of the treatment of paraplegic patients, which are still valid today. Guttmann organized the Paralympics in Stoke Mandeville in the 1950s as part of his effort to promote the social reintegration of his patients. Currently, this sports event is held after the "normal" Olympic Games at the same site.

Loss of function occurs in specific muscle groups depending on the location of the injury (▶Table 7.3). Flaccid paralysis and loss of all reflex activity below the level of injury occur immediately after the injury.

All paraplegic patients suffer from deconditioning syndrome (Chapter 2), and they all can benefit from therapeutic exercise. Learning a sport is generally recommended to paraplegic patients at the latest during their time in the rehabilitation clinic. Regardless of the level of the injury, almost all patients are able to perform adapted strength and endurance training. Intensive training, particularly in patients with incomplete paraplegia, can result in an increase in strength even years later. However, one must also remember that the plasticity of the cord spinal is very limited or even negligible. Recent studies in rats by van den Brand et al[414] proved that with electrochemical stimulation and intensive robot-assisted treadmill training, rats could even learn to walk again. The applicapibilty of this method to humans is still unclear.

Adapted endurance training is important for paraplegic patients, as it helps to stabilize and improve the circulatory situation. The focus in strength training is to achieve sufficient upright posture of the trunk.

> **Note**
>
> In both endurance and strength training, it is important that the patients do not become overheated, as their heat regulation can be impaired.

Patients with traumatic paraplegia, even those with a very high injury, can pursue sports activities, such as wheelchair rugby, athletic disciplines, or winter sports. Patients who practice sports at a high level may even train up to 10 hours, for example, in a training camp. A well, thought-out training plan can avoid overtaxing the patients.

Paraplegic patients can use all the strength and endurance equipment that patients in wheelchairs use. Lat-pull machines, cycling trainers, and upper body ergometers are particularly suitable strength training devices. Other equipment can only be used if the patients are able to affect the transfer, and the equipment provides sufficient support for the safe training of the patients. The important thing is to combine strength training with endurance training and to have patients practice standing during therapeutic exercise if they do not stand at home. The balance trainer can be used for dynamic stance training (Chapter 6.4.1, ▶Fig. 7.10).

> **Note**
>
> All paraplegic patients should be encouraged to participate in a sport to minimize the negative effects of lack of movement.

Table 7.3 Location of injury and affected muscle groups.

Level of injury	Affected muscle groups
C1	Short muscles of the neck
C4	Diaphragm
C5	Biceps brachii
C6	Brachioradialis, extensor carpi radialis
C7	Triceps brachii
C8	Long extensors of the fingers, thumb extensors
T1	Hypothenar, intrinsic muscles of the hand
L1/2	Psoas, hip adductors
L3	Quadriceps
L4	Tibialis anterior, vastus medialis
L5	Extensor hallucis longus, extensor digitorum brevis
S1	Triceps surae, peroneus muscles, gluteus maximus
S2/3	Flexor digitorum brevis
S4/5	External anal sphincter

7.6 Craniocerebral Trauma

After stroke, the second most common cause of severe disabilities with immobility is craniocerebral trauma.

> **Definition** [ ]
>
> "Craniocerebral trauma is the result of a forceful impact that has led to functional impairment and/or injury of the brain and can be associated with a contusion of or injury to the scalp, cranium, blood vessels, brain tissue, and/or dura mater."[15]

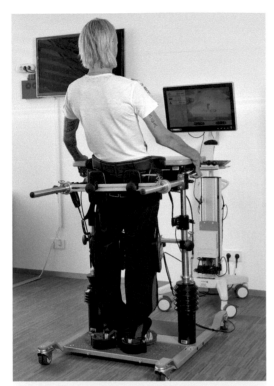

Fig. 7.10 Dynamic stance training with the balance trainer.

The incidence of craniocerebral trauma is approximately 330 per 100,000 per year.[335] About 90% of all cases are slight craniocerebral injuries, and approximately 5% can be classified as severe craniocerebral trauma. Severe craniocerebral trauma is present when the initial score according to the Glasgow Coma Scale is 8 to 3 points, or the posttraumatic impairment of consciousness persists longer than 24 hours, and/or brainstem symptoms occur.[399] The incidence of severe craniocerebral trauma in Germany is estimated to be about 15 to 20 patients per 100,000 per year.[15]

The outcome of severe craniocerebral trauma is influenced by many factors, including age, initial score on the Glasgow Coma Scale, and elevated intracranial pressure. In spite of significant advances in intensive care and decreasing mortality, the prognosis for patients with severe craniocerebral trauma remains unfavorable. About 40 to 50% of patients die, 2 to 14% of patients survive in a permanent vegetative state (Apallic syndrome),[201] 10 to 30% remain severely disabled, and 17 to 20% remain moderately disabled. Only 7 to 27%

of patients with severe craniocerebral trauma recover well.[252] In one-third of all patients with craniocerebral trauma, the injury occurred before the age of 30.

The treatment of patients with craniocerebral trauma follows the approach used with stroke patients. A major difference between patients with craniocerebral trauma and stroke patients is their age and thus their cardiovascular situation. Patients with craniocerebral trauma may exhibit a deconditioning syndrome as a result of an extended posttraumatic coma (Chapter 3). Patients with craniocerebral trauma benefit from training in the same way as stroke patients.

7.7 Cerebral Palsy

Children with cerebral palsy suffer from motor and cognitive disabilities. The goal of therapy with these children is to maximize their functional abilities. Children with cerebral palsy should begin training as early as possible, and training should be very intensive. Taking pauses is important for consolidating the motor memory. Strength training has been shown to benefit children with cerebral palsy and does not exacerbate spasticity.[76,107]

Gorter et al[149] showed that two weekly 30-minute sessions of circuit training at four stations over a period of 9 weeks improved endurance and functional walking ability in children with cerebral palsy.

Impaired walking ability is one of the most common problems that cerebral palsy patients face in daily life. This problem stems from an initial lack of strength in the musculature. As time passes, these patients develop extension spasticity of varying intensity as a compensatory mechanism to allow locomotion. The age at which children should participate in a therapeutic exercise regime must be answered on a case-by-case basis.

Treadmill training with a body weight–support system improves the walking speed. Children with particularly severe disabilities benefit from this training.[433,62] A Lokomat for children was first marketed in 2006 that allowed an intensive gait training to be conducted with children aged 4 years and older. The results of a study by Borggräfe et al[39] demonstrated significantly increased walking distance and walking speed following robot-assisted treadmill training. The intervention included 3 weeks of training for 10 to 45 minutes conducted four times a week.

The introduction of virtual reality computer programs suitable for children can increase repetition. This can fulfill one of the most important and basic principles of motor learning. All areas of therapeutic exercise can be exploited for adolescents or adults who had infantile cerebral palsy.

Many children or adolescents with cerebral palsy have no motivation to undergo physical therapy. Aside from its therapeutic benefits, therapeutic exercise provides these patients an opportunity to engage in physical activity with persons of comparable age. Adolescents should be watched closely to ensure they do not use too many weights. Training should follow the Borg scale for these patients as well. Aside from endurance and strength training, patients with cerebral palsy also need to work on agility, balance, and stretching ability.

7.8 Neuromuscular Disorders

The collective term "neuromuscular disorders" refers to a heterogeneous group of diseases. The common point among them is the pathology of a component of the motor unit. This motor unit is a functional unit consisting of a motor neuron with its axon that via the anterior root and peripheral nerve supplies the muscle fibers via the motor endplate.[370] The essential common feature of neuromuscular disorders is muscle weakness, which is usually progressive (▶Fig. 7.11). A single classification system follows the location of the disorder (▶Fig. 7.12).

7.8.1 General Notes

The primary goal of therapy in patients with neuromuscular disorders is to preserve walking ability. Patients with neuromuscular disorders typically suffer increasing scoliosis, contractures, and decreasing respiratory function once they lose the ability to walk.[212] Contractures are a typical problem of patients with neuromuscular disorders.[258] Therefore, the entire therapy should focus on the prevention and prophylaxis of contractures.[371]

In recent years, a trend toward greater activity in therapy even with patients with neuromuscular disorders has initiated. Therapeutic exercise is only one part of the rehabilitation of these patients. The use of orthoses and/or walking aids can preserve walking ability longer. Properly supplying

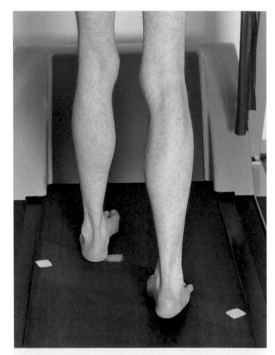

Fig. 7.11 Neuromuscular disorder.

these aids to patients with Duchenne's muscular dystrophy can prolong their walking ability by 2 to 3 years.[166] Appropriate physical therapy is also necessary to minimize sequelae.

The majority of neuromuscular disorders are slowly or rapidly progressive, and muscle function deteriorates over time. This means that the training program must be continually adapted to the patient according to the progression of the disorder. Therapeutic exercise is unable to halt the progression of the disease. Also, no studies exist that have examined the long-term effect of this form of therapy on the patients' life situation.[212]

Given the lack of such studies, it is not currently possible to make any general recommendations about the intensity, frequency, and duration of the training intervention in patients with neuromuscular disorders. The exercise tolerance of these patients depends on many factors, such as the etiology and progression of the disease, involvement of organs (for example, cardiovascular involvement), and the severity of the muscle weakness.[212] The level of serum creatine kinase has not proven to be a reliable indicator. As a result, exercise tolerance must be

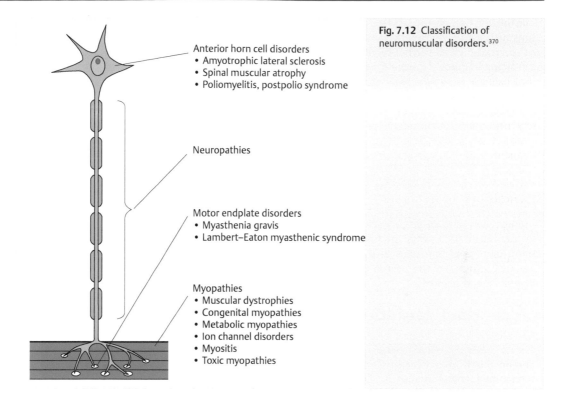

Fig. 7.12 Classification of neuromuscular disorders.[370]

Anterior horn cell disorders
• Amyotrophic lateral sclerosis
• Spinal muscular atrophy
• Poliomyelitis, postpolio syndrome

Neuropathies

Motor endplate disorders
• Myasthenia gravis
• Lambert–Eaton myasthenic syndrome

Myopathies
• Muscular dystrophies
• Congenital myopathies
• Metabolic myopathies
• Ion channel disorders
• Myositis
• Toxic myopathies

determined for each individual patient by carefully increasing the requirements. Criteria for the limit of exercise tolerance may include the occurrence of myalgia or overly long recuperative pauses.[392] Training should be conducted at a level below the limit of exercise tolerance determined in this manner.

7.8.2 Recommendations for Endurance Training

Patients with neuromuscular disorders should receive individual or group training to improve their endurance. The proper target heart rate should be determined by exercise ergometry.[442] However, note that no studies exist that demonstrate that the target heart rate determined in healthy subjects is also valid for patients with neuromuscular disorders.[212] In the case of a possible cardiac involvement, ECG monitoring is indicated during ergometry, and the endurance training should be performed with pulse monitoring. Training should occur within the aerobic threshold.[212]

> **Note**
>
> A training frequency of three times a week can be assumed as a guideline value for endurance training. Interval training of 2 to 3 minutes with a pause of at least 1 minute over a period of 15 to 30 minutes appears to be suitable.[442]

7.8.3 Recommendations for Strength Training

Training should be conducted at below the maximum exertion level and should reflect the clinical symptoms. Training with maximum resistance is not beneficial to these patients. Aitkens et al[5] showed that training at even 20 to 40% of the maximum strength can have a positive effect on the strength for patients with slowly progressive neuromuscular disorders. Kilmer et al[207] also found positive effects of maximum strength training in patients with slowly progressive neuromuscular disorders but also worsening in some cases.

However, the improvements were not greater than those achieved with strength training at 20 to 40% of the maximum strength. One recommendation for training frequency is three times a week with a 1-day pause between the sessions.

No conclusive studies exist on the combination of endurance and strength training in patients with neuromuscular disorders.[212]

7.8.4 Motor Neuron Disorders (Anterior Horn Cell Disorders)

In motor neuron disorders, muscle weakness and atrophy occur as a result of increasing loss of motor neurons in the spinal cord and brainstem. The most common motor neuron disorder is amyotrophic lateral sclerosis.

Amyotrophic Lateral Sclerosis

> **Definition**   [ ]
>
> Amyotrophic lateral sclerosis (ALS) is a progressive degenerative motor system disorder of the upper and lower motor neurons.

Except for the rare hereditary form of the disease, the cause of ALS is not known. The prevalence of the disease appears to be increasing worldwide. According to Carter,[55] its worldwide prevalence is about 5 to 7 per 100,000 individuals. Age at the onset is between 40 and 60 years; men are affected 1.5 times more often than women. The risk of smokers contracting the disease appears to be three times higher.[139]

The course of the disorder varies greatly between individuals. Life expectancy is reduced with the 5-year survival rate of around 28%. Ten to twenty percent of patients with ALS survive longer than 10 years after the diagnosis. It exclusively affects the motor nervous system; the vegetative system is not affected. This means that touch sensation, pain and temperature sensation, sight, hearing, smell and taste, bladder and bowel function, and especially cognitive ability remain intact.

The motor system, which controls the muscles and steers movements, is affected both in its central components (brain, brainstem, and spinal cord) and peripheral ones (anterior horn cells). Except for the rare familial form of the disease (5–10% of all cases), ALS is not a hereditary disorder.

Aside from palliative care, adapted and properly guided strength training can achieve a positive effect.[99,71] Light endurance training and adapted physical therapy to avoid contractures, improvement of general cardiovascular endurance, and mobilization of the ribcage to improve respiratory function are necessary. According to the Borg scale, after training, patients with ALS should feel pleasantly tired but not exhausted. Two or three training sessions a week under proper medical supervision are recommended. Patients should also perform a daily exercise program at home; swimming and water gymnastics are recommended.

> **Note**
>
> Overly intensive strength training leading to exhaustion or even muscle pain should be avoided.[80]

Training both the upper and lower extremities with a cycling trainer is recommended for patients with ALS. A standing frame that is also conductive to mobile standing, such as the balance trainer shown here, is recommended. It is important to carefully instruct the patients to follow the Borg scale. Patients with ALS should train to improve function and not to strengthen their muscles. Patients with ALS under training must be informed about the warning signs of overexertion. Overexertion may occur when the patient experiences a feeling of weakness within 30 minutes of training or muscle pain occurs 24–48 hours after exertion. Muscle cramps, a sensation of heaviness in the arms and legs, and persistent shortness of breath are also signs of overexertion. Patients must learn to pay attention to these signs of overexertion.

Spinal Muscular Atrophy

The progressive spinal muscular atrophies (SMAs) are a clinically and genetically heterogeneous group of disorders that occur as a result of the selective degeneration of anterior horn cells and the motor nuclei of the brainstem.[435] Spinal muscular atrophies are classified in three grades according to their severity and age of manifestation. The most severe form is SMA type 1, known as Werdnig–Hoffmann disease. Most children die before the second year of life. SMA type 2 is also referred to as an intermediate form that manifests itself between the age of 8 and 18 months. The children are able to sit up but unable to walk and life expectancy is 10 to 20 years. SMA type 3, known as Kugelberg-Welander disease, begins after the age of 18 months but before the age of 30 years. There is only slight muscular atrophy, and life expectancy is hardly shorter than normal. Therapeutic exercise is not possible in SMA type 1 and 2. Patients with SMA type 3 should undergo careful endurance training in therapeutic exercise. Many of the patients feel that isometric strength training is helpful in improving mobility and coordination.[451]

Post Polio Syndrome

Post polio syndrome is defined as the occurrence of symptoms after an asymptomatic period of at least 15 years in a patient who previously suffered from poliomyelitis. As acute anterior poliomyelitis is often asymptomatic or only minimally symptomatic, the exact number of infected persons is not known. It is assumed that about 50% of persons infected with polio develop post polio syndrome. The diagnosis of post polio syndrome is made by exclusion. It is thought to be caused by the degeneration of previously damaged motor neurons.[212] A few studies have demonstrated the efficacy of strength training.[3,4,59,109] Also, studies exist on endurance training of patients with post polio syndrome.[200,217] These studies have been evaluated differently due to flaws in their methodology.[211] The EFNS task force has evaluated strength training in these patients positively regard the evidence as insufficient.[115,70]

Training aspects:
- There is a risk of overexertion; training should be regulated.
- Endurance training is good for optimizing cardiovascular exercise tolerance.
- Strength training is recommended to improve neuromuscular coordination.[376]
- Aerobic training is recommended, as are pauses between exercises and free days between the three weekly training sessions.
- Muscle soreness and persistent exhaustion should be avoided.
- Training should begin at 20% of maximum exercise capacity.[283]

7.8.5 Neuropathy

Neuropathy is a collective term for various disorders of the peripheral nervous system that are attributable to a functional impairment or pathologic change. Mononeuropathy refers to the involvement of only one nerve, whereas polyneuropathy denotes an involvement of several nerves. Hereditary neuropathies are clinically and genetically heterogeneous groups of disorders of the peripheral nerves. There are many forms of hereditary motor and sensory neuropathies that are of negligible clinical importance due to the small number of individual forms. No data are available on the prevalence and incidence of hereditary motor and sensory neuropathies that develop symptoms in adulthood. Charcot–Marie–Tooth disease (peroneal muscular atrophy) is the most common form of hereditary neuropathy. The hereditary neuropathies are usually slowly progressive disorders.

Hereditary Motor and Sensory Neuropathy, Charcot–Marie–Tooth Disease

Patients with Charcot–Marie–Tooth (CMT) disease exhibit characteristic symmetrical muscular atrophy and paresis in the upper and lower extremities, absent reflexes, foot deformities, and disturbed gait (▶Fig. 7.13). Sensory deficits of varying severity are present. The muscular atrophy begins in the distal lower extremities and later spreads to the upper extremities as the disease progresses. The disorder is usually slowly progressive. Patients seem to adapt well in daily life, although apparently, they suffer more. Affected persons require more than twice as long as healthy persons to put on a T-shirt or walk 10 meters.[304]

In addition to physical therapy to manage or prevent the foot deformity and muscle contracture, a

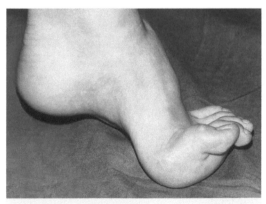

Fig. 7.13 Typical foot deformity in a patient with CMT.

regime of therapeutic exercise is helpful and should be conducted regularly. Strength training is also recommended in addition to endurance training. Lindeman et al [238] demonstrated that strength training at a frequency of three times a week over a period of 24 weeks shows positive effects in patients with CMT. Chetlin et al showed that strength training three times a week over a period of 12 weeks has a positive effect on strength and the activities of daily life in both male and female patients.[63] We may conclude from this that patients with CMT benefit from both endurance and strength training. Patients with CMT also benefit from focused stretching of the calf musculature.[106] As with all neuromuscular disorders, both the endurance and strength training must be adapted to the patient's specific condition. The important thing is that patients with CMT are properly supplied with the necessary walking aids. Patients should also receive occupational therapy consultation and treatment.[304]

Peripheral Neuropathy

Polyneuropathies from other causes are more significant than the hereditary motor and sensory neuropathies. These include polyneuropathies due to diabetes, alcoholism, drug toxicity, and inflammatory processes. In the western world, diabetes is the most common cause of neuropathy.[387] In spite of this, the prevalence and incidence of the disorder are not known. The only certainty is that there is a positive correlation between the incidence and the duration of the disorder.

The treatment of peripheral neuropathy involves the management of the underlying disorder and the preservation of mobility and strength. This indicates that therapeutic exercise must focus on training strength and walking with the two factors, speed and walking endurance. Balducci et al[16] demonstrated that the development of diabetic polyneuropathy can be delayed with regular aerobic training. Alternating between strength training and coordination training is also recommended, as are endurance training and appropriate sports.[120,322,408] Three weeks of specific balance training and training distal power leads to a significant improvement in many measured parameters (single-leg stance, functional reach, tandem stance).

Therapeutic exercise is an excellent means of training balance in patients with neuropathy. The important thing for patients is to train balance with their eyes closed. To achieve it, the patient must be able to train in a situation with no risk of falling. The Posturomed and the Zeptor are very suitable machines for balance training. To prevent compensation as a result of visual feedback, the patient must train with the eyes closed or while turning the head from side-to-side or up and down. The therapist should ensure that the patient does not fix his or her gaze (ballerina effect). Neuropathy patients can also train endurance and strength in therapeutic exercise programs without having to fear overexertion.

Acute Inflammatory Demyelinating Polyradiculoneuropathy or Guillain–Barré Syndrome

Acute inflammatory demyelinating polyradiculoneuropathy is an inflammatory disorder of the peripheral nerves characterized by infiltration of the nerve tissue by lymphocytes and macrophages that leads to destruction of the myelin sheath of the nerve fibers. Guillain–Barré syndrome (GBS) is an acute polyneuropathy that can be treated with plasmapheresis and intravenous immunglobulins. GBS can also affect the cranial nerves; about 20% of patients with GBS develop muscular respiratory insufficiency within a few days.

To avoid secondary problems, patients with GBS should be brought into an upright position for training by the physician. Endurance and strength training should also begin as soon as possible. According to a study by Forssberg,[127] 12% of patients with GBS were still limited in their activities of daily life after 2 years, and 17% had not returned to work. One year after the onset of the disease, 50% of the patients had limitations in the leisure activities and 30% suffered limitations at work.[28] Fatigue is a major problem for patients with GBS, as approximately 80%suffer from the syndrome; moreover, fatigue responds poorly to medications.[304] Garssen et al[142] demonstrated that aerobic endurance training had a positive effect on fatigue in patients with GBS.

Critical Illness Polyneuropathy, Critical Illness Myopathy

Critical illness polyneuropathy (CIP) and critical illness myopathy (CIM) are functional impairments that can occur in isolation or together in an acquired weakness syndrome in the intensive care unit.

Mertens described the occurrence of polyneuropathy in comatose patients in 1963.[453] He reported on six patients in whom often disseminated, asymmetrical neuropathy occurred. Bolton et al defined CIP as a symptom complex in its own right in 1984. They found primarily distal symmetrical axonal damage and regarded difficulty in adapting to the withdrawal of assisted ventilation as an early leading clinical sign.[189] The pathophysiology of CIM has yet to be explained. The prevalence of CIP is probably higher than previously suspected. According to a prospective study, 35% of patients with sepsis and multiple organ failure have polyneuropathy.[194]

The underlying disorder is not the decisive factor for the development of CIP; the decisive factor is the time that these patients have spent in the intensive care unit. Clinical signs include generalized muscular weakness with weakened or absent intrinsic reflexes. There is no known specific therapy. In therapeutic exercise, the focus is on carefully strengthening the muscles with additional endurance training.

7.8.6 Disorders of Neuromuscular Transmission

Myasthenia Gravis

Myasthenia gravis is a chronic autoimmune disorder of the neuromuscular synapses with loss of acetylcholine receptors.[360] The prevalence of myasthenia gravis lies between 2.5 and 10 per 100,000 individuals and most often manifests itself between the age of 20 and 40 and between the age of 60 and 70. The ratio of male to female cases is 3:2.[183]

The cardinal symptom of myasthenia gravis is weakness in the striated muscles that increases with exertion and also fluctuates. Most patients find this fluctuating weakness to be a significant impairment in the activities of daily life and thus a reduction in their quality of life. With good medication, many patients remain largely asymptomatic. The residual symptoms can be reduced with physical and sports therapy.[441] Wolfsegger et al demonstrated that patients with myasthenia gravis had lower endurance than a comparable control group. Endurance loads up to 4 mmol/L and muscular endurance loads up to 60% of the maximum contractions are well tolerated. However, the extent to which training is possible with these patients remains to be demonstrated.

Eaton–Lambert Syndrom, Lambert–Eaton Myasthenic Syndrome

At a prevalence of about 0.35 per 100,000 individuals, Lambert–Eaton myasthenic syndrome is far less common that myasthenia gravis. The syndrome is an immune-mediated condition with formation of antibodies, which attack the voltage-gated P/Q type calcium channels. The result is an impaired release of acetylcholine at cholinergic synapses of the motor and autonomic nerve systems. This leads to proximally pronounced muscular weakness. Maximum power generation is delayed several seconds, and progressive exertion leads to muscle fatigue. Primarily, the lower extremities and trunk are affected.

Typical signs include weakness and rapid onset of fatigue when walking, standing from a low sitting position, and climbing stairs. Walking distance can be greatly reduced (less than 100 meters), and intrinsic reflexes are reduced.

7.8.7 Myopathies

Myopathies are an etiologically heterogeneous group of muscular disorders. Most myopathies are characterized by proximally pronounced paresis and atrophy. Paresis of the entire muscular system may occur in the later course of the disease. Agonists and antagonists are affected to differing degrees so that deformities and contractures can develop. Where the legs are affected, the patient's ability to stand and walk gets impaired.

Muscular Dystrophy

Muscular dystrophies are genetic disorders of the muscles. Increasing deterioration of muscle fibers occurs as the disease progresses. The striated musculature is replaced with fatty fibrous degenerative tissue. There is a broad range of clinical manifestations. Duchenne muscular dystrophy and Becker muscular dystrophy are caused by derangement or absence of the X-linked recessive gene product dystrophin, a structural protein. The absence of dystrophin appears to destabilize the muscle membrane, thus making the muscle fibers increasingly susceptible to mechanical stress.[212] Note that the patient's exercise tolerance is decreased when the heart is affected.

Sveen et al[391] demonstrated in a study the efficacy of endurance training with Becker muscular dystrophy. They found an improvement in performance after 12 weeks of training without an increase in creatine kinase (CK) values, and they also measured increased strength in the musculature. Continuing training over a period of 1 year did not show any negative effect with respect to CK values or with muscle biopsies. In 2013, Sveen et al demonstrated that even moderate strength training was able to improve strength and endurance in Becker muscular dystrophy and limb–girdle muscular dystrophy. The study reported improvement with both low-intensity training and high-intensity training. However, one candidate had to interrupt high-intensity training because of the muscle soreness.[391,390]

Limb–girdle muscular dystrophies are a group of muscular dystrophies that can affect either sex and whose initial symptoms appear in the shoulder girdle or pelvic girdle. The term, limb–girdle muscular dystrophy, is used internationally for this group of disorders. A distinction is made between autosomal dominant and autosomal recessive forms of limb–girdle muscular dystrophy. Both forms of limb–girdle muscular dystrophy can be further subdivided according to the location of gene defect. Several studies have documented the benefit of strength training and endurance training in slowly progressive muscular dystrophies. In rapidly progressive forms, there is a risk that excessively intensive training may cause additional damage. In every type of muscular dystrophy, training must be planned on an individual basis, and both therapist and patient must be alerted to the signs of overexertion.

Congenital Myopathies

Congenital myopathies are also genetic muscular diseases that begin in early childhood, sometimes even in newborns. The clinical course tends to be static. The children are hypotonic, have difficulty drinking, and can exhibit skeletal deformities. Some congenital myopathies remain unchanged over their clinical course or show slight improvement.

Metabolic Myopathies

A muscular metabolic derangement leads to metabolic myopathy, a genetic disorder. However, the symptoms often appear only in early adulthood. Pompe's disease is a glycogen storage disorder that follows an autosomal recessive pattern of inheritance and manifests itself especially in the muscles. For this reason, it is regarded as a myopathy. The disorder can occur at any age. In infantile Pompe's disease, the first symptoms can occur at the age of about 2 months. The infants die in the first year of life from heart failure. Late-onset disease in adolescents and adult patients does not follow a uniform clinical course and is therefore difficult to predict. Muscular weakness occurs, especially in the respiratory and trunk musculature. The clinical course depends on the duration of the disease, not the age of the patient. There are indications that endurance training in combination with a protein-rich diet is helpful.[373]

Ion Channel Disorders

Ion channel disorders are a heterogeneous group of hereditary disorders usually characterized by episodic clinical symptoms of impaired stimulation of the musculature or nervous system. These disorders include the myotonias and the periodic paralyses that do not lead to increasing loss of muscle cells.[230]

The physician must determine the extent to which training may be helpful or harmful, as some of these disorders respond negatively to physical exertion.

Myositis

Myositis is the generic term for a rare heterogeneous group of acquired inflammatory muscle disorders that can lead to progressively limited motion and increasing morbidity by the involvement of organs other than the muscles. Myositides are acquired autoimmune diseases of muscle and include polymyositis, dermatomyositis, and inclusion body myositis.

These myositis syndromes are rare and very heterogeneous. Therefore, hardly any studies exist on the efficacy of medications or other interventions.[89] Women develop polymyositis and dermatomyositis about twice as often as men, whereas men develop dermatomyositis about three times as often as women. The age at onset is around 18 years and older for polymyositis. For dermatomyositis, there are two age cohorts, 5 to 15 years and 45 to 65 years. The age of onset for inclusion body myositis patients is over 50 years.

The pareses in patients with polymyositis and dermatomyositis tend to be more proximal than distal and are symmetrical. Patients with inclusion body myositis exhibit proximal and distal pareses equally often. The distribution is asymmetrical. The flexors of the fingers and the foot dorsiflexors are often particularly involved. Pronounced atrophy can be observed in these patients. Neuropathies are frequent comorbidities in inclusion body myositis. Polymyositis and dermatomyositis are often associated with myocarditis, interstitial lung disease, malignancies, vasculitis, and other systemic diseases such as collage disease.[89] All three forms are characterized by muscle weakness, whereas sensory function and intrinsic reflexes are spared. Approximately 50% of patients also develop pain in the muscles and/or joints. In the advanced stages of all three forms, the swallowing, respiratory, and neck muscles can be involved as well.

A few studies come to the conclusion that patients can benefit from moderate physical training with a cycle ergometer and stepper. However, these studies only included a very small number of patients with myositis.[8,431]

Toxic Myopathies

Toxic myopathies are caused by ingestion of external substances. The most common toxic substances are medications and alcohol. Toxic myopathies can manifest themselves as muscle pain, muscle weakness, or even as rhabdomyolysis.[162]

7.9 Hereditary Spastic Paraplegia

This is also known as hereditary spastic paraparesis. Hereditary spastic paraplegia is not a disease but a group of clinically heterogeneous hereditary disorders. Hereditary spastic paraplegia is characterized by spastic weakness of the lower extremities. There are two different degrees of severity:
- The uncomplicated forms, which aside from spasticity in the legs, include only slight sensory deficits in the calves and feet and slight problems with bladder emptying.
- The second group of spinal paraplegia disorders include those with rare complicated clinical courses associated with peripheral nerve impairments, epilepsy, dementia, ataxia (impaired voluntary movements), or disorders of the eye.

The symptoms usually occur between the age of 20 and 40 but can also begin much earlier or much later. Patients experience increasing stiffness in the legs, followed by an unsteady gait and balance problems. Spastic paraplegia typically includes extension spasticity of the legs.

The disorder is slowly progressive. Rapid deterioration or rapid spontaneous improvement suggests other disorders. About one-third of all patients develop disturbed micturition with incontinence and an imperative urge to urinate. As hereditary spastic paraplegia is a genetically transmitted disorder, no causal therapy is possible. Therefore, the focus is on symptomatic treatment. In addition to medications to influence the spasticity, physical therapy and thus therapeutic exercise are the treatments of first choice. As with all other disorders that involve spasticity, reducing spasticity while simultaneously training a functional task is the means of choice. Gait training reduces spasticity while simultaneously training the muscles needed for walking. Severely impaired patients with spastic paraplegia can benefit from the use of lococycling trainers.

7.10 Severely Impaired Patients and Therapeutic Exercise

"Therapeutic exercise" and "severely impaired neurologic patients" would appear at first glance to be irreconcilable entities, posing more questions than answers.

When do we refer to neurologic patients as "severely impaired"? When the patient can no longer walk? Or when he or she can no longer perform activities of daily life alone?

When can or should we speak of training or therapeutic exercise? Does therapeutic exercise require that the patient actively train on many pieces of equipment? Or does therapeutic exercise for severely impaired patients mean nothing more than standing in a standing device or a session with a cycling trainer?

> **Note**
>
> These questions require a pragmatic approach: As soon as a severely impaired patient practices or trains at his or her tolerance limit, we can consider employing therapeutic exercise. One should take into account if this exercise is structured and adapted to the patient's needs and is performed with the objective of improving basic motor skills according to a plan.

8 Organizational Matters

8.1 Planning Training

Optimal planning is the basis for achieving a good result with therapeutic exercise regimes for neurologic patients. What is true for therapeutic exercise in general also applies to therapeutic exercise with neurologic patients: Before beginning the therapy, it is crucial to obtain comprehensive findings that will necessarily differ from the physiotherapist's findings. Aside from functional impairments and impaired abilities, this comprehensive report should also include conditioned abilities, social setting, emotional states (emotion and motivation), and cognitive requirements. These findings are obtained when the history is taken, and various suitable tests and assessments are performed.

The goals of therapy (short, middle, and long term) are defined in cooperation with the patient on the basis of these data. Once these goals are clearly formulated, a training plan takes shape that forms the basis of therapeutic exercise. As the therapeutic exercise regime is put into practice, the current results at any given time are always compared with the targets, which are accordingly modified in applicable cases. Training with neurologic patients is not fundamentally different from training with other patients. The decisive factors in determining the training parameters include the respective diagnoses, severity of the disability, patient's goals, and the rehabilitation prognosis. Training parameters for the respective clinical pictures are discussed in Chapter 7. Note that these must be adapted to the patient's specific capabilities and daily ups and downs.

In the literature, modified Karvonen's formula together with the Borg scale is currently the preferred method for controlling endurance training. Using the parameters of maximum strength for planning strength training is not always feasible or advisable with many neurologic patients. Nonetheless, it is repeatedly stated that strength training should be performed at about 40% of the maximum strength.

> **Note**
>
> One can use the Borg scale as a guide when planning training for patients with neurologic deficits. This will also aid in adapting training to the daily or hourly fluctuations in exertion.

However, training for neurologic patients cannot be pressed into a mold. Patients' problems vary greatly between individuals and can depend on the specific day or time of the day. Especially in patients with disorders of the neuromuscular junction, the exertion must be finely adapted to the patient's shape on that specific day to avoid damage to the musculature.

Well-planned pauses constitute an important requirement for making therapeutic exercise a useful complement to the rehabilitation of patients with neurologic deficits. These pauses must be observed, especially in patients with multiple sclerosis and neuromuscular disorders.

A pause does not mean that the patient sits ideal. On the contrary, other muscle groups should be trained at this time or the patient can use this time to learn new compensation strategies and motion sequences by observation.

> **Note**
>
> The timing of pauses always depends on the patient's state of health. However, the pauses should not be too long. The following rule of thumb applies:
> - For simple motions, the pause should be about half as long as the time required for the exercise.
> - For complex motions, the pause should be about as long as the time required for the exercise.

8.2 Personnel Requirements

> **Note**
>
> In neurologic therapeutic exercise, patients may only be entrusted to the care of therapists who have appropriate experience in the care and supervision of neurologic patients.

Personnel investment into therapeutic exercise is definitely measurably higher due to the patients' various disabilities compared with patients with orthopaedic and postsurgical conditions. Patients, especially with cognitive difficulties require an enormous investment. The greatest personnel investment is required at the beginning of training and while learning new exercises.

Physical therapists in therapeutic exercise must be familiar with the appropriate equipment and must be well versed in the fundamentals of training research and motor learning. Sports researchers and sports therapists must be trained in the basics of neurologic pathology. Moreover, they must have a fundamental understanding of obtaining physical therapy findings in neurologic patients.

Regular training of all persons involved in therapeutic exercise is essential to assure quality care. To maintain the standard and quality of care for the individual patients, only a few "new" patients should be admitted to existing groups at any particular time. This group should represent a good mix of slightly and severely impaired patients. It is always important that all patients actually receive the attention and supervision they require.

Patients must be well supervised so that they receive the maximum benefit from therapeutic exercise. The investment of supervision of neurologic patients in therapeutic exercise is definitely higher than in the musculoskeletal or cardiovascular training. One way to facilitate the supervision of neurologic patients is to utilize training devices equipped with a chip function that automatically accesses presets and training parameters. However, these devices are incapable of automatically detecting fluctuations in the performance of patients. Even when patients utilize units with automatic settings, these must be monitored by trained professionals.

With myriad of machines employed in therapeutic exercise, it is difficult or impossible to maneuver a wheelchair directly into the unit. This infers that it is often necessary to assist patients into using the machine. Caregivers must be trained and able to perform these transfers.

It is also imperative to ensure that the seats of the respective machines are large enough to provide comfortable, secure seating even for severely impaired patients. In larger facilities with a high volume of patients, it is essential to ensure that enough caregivers are available to provide assistance as required. The therapeutic exercise rooms in rehabilitation facilities and hospitals should remain open as long as possible for therapeutic reasons. To allow patients who are already independent to train, facilities should also offer certain training times under the supervision of a staff member who need not be a therapist. Patients who train at these times must have the approval of their physician or therapist for such training.

8.3 Required Facilities

The facilities required for therapeutic exercise in neurology are no different from those used by orthopaedic patients. The important factor is to allow enough space between the individual units so that wheelchair patients can conveniently maneuver up to the devices and transfer into them.

The choice of devices is crucial and must be adapted to the patient's needs (Chapter 6). It is a good idea to number the devices and use these numbers in the training plans of patients so that they can easily access them. In the rehabilitation facility or clinic, the attending physician, occasionally at the request of the therapist, refers the patient to therapeutic exercise. Outpatient facilities necessitate a different form of organization, as training on equipment is often not covered by health insurance funds. If no way exists to bill the use of therapeutic exercise machines to statutory health insurance funds, patients are forced to pay for this service themselves.

9 Tests and Assessments

9.1 Tests for Neurorehabilitation

Numerous tests and assessments are available for all clinical pictures and symptoms (▶Fig. 9.1, ▶Fig. 9.2, ▶Fig. 9.3, ▶Fig. 9.4, ▶Fig. 9.5, ▶Fig. 9.6, and ▶Fig. 9.7). In many clinics and rehabilitation facilities, these tests are stipulated by the management. In therapy centers, these tests are often insufficiently utilized to critically assess the impact of therapy. However, even therapists working on an outpatient basis get used to the fact that the health insurance funds require positive evidence of the progress of therapy. This is what scientifically verified tests and assessments are for.

The tests presented here (▶Table 9.1) can usually be performed quickly and easily even in an outpatient setting. Most tests and the appropriate evaluation instructions are available on the internet or via the literature cited. The list of tests in ▶Table 9.1 is neither comprehensive nor exclusive. Alternatives are also available in many areas. However, it is important that the tests are validated.

In therapeutic exercise in neurology, it is necessary to determine the patient's function and document the patient's progress. A large number of test methods are available for this purpose.

> **Note**
>
> These tests must be valid, practicable, reliable, and sensitive.

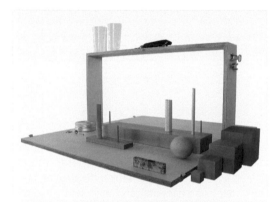

Fig. 9.1 Action Research Arm Test (ARAT).

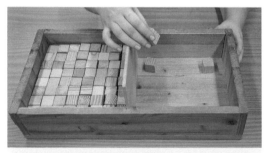

Fig. 9.2 Box and Block Test (BBT).

Dynamic Gait Index		
Patient name		DOB:
Tester		
Walking aids		Date:
Item		Point score
1	Walking on a level surface 20 m	
2	Walking with speed change, 5 m normal, 5 m fast, 5 m slow	
3	Walking while turning head right and left	
4	Walking while looking up and down	
5	Walking and turning 180 degrees	
6	Walking over obstacles	
7	Walking around obstacles to the left and right	
8	Climbing stairs	
Total points (maximum 24)		

Fig. 9.3 Dynamic Gait Index (DGI).

▶**Validity.** The term, validity, means that the test has been confirmed and is internationally recognized.

▶**Practicability.** Practicability of a test examines the necessity of special devices or softwares, efficiency of the training investment for the testers, and the amount of time invested in the test itself.

▶**Reliability.** Another word for reliability is invariability, which means that the measured values correspond to the actual value. The test should produce the same result when repeated by the same examiner, and should produce the same result when performed by two different therapists.

▶**Responsiveness.** Responsiveness refers to sensitivity and addresses the sensitivity of the test to measure even small improvements in rehabilitation.

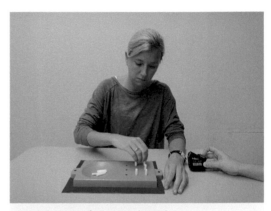

Fig. 9.5 Nine Hole Peg Test (NHPT).

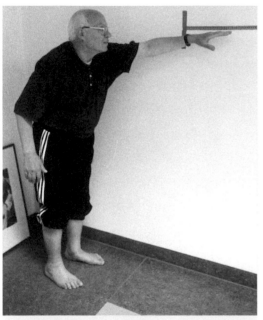

Fig. 9.4 Functional Reach Test.

Fig. 9.6 Wolf Motor Function Test.

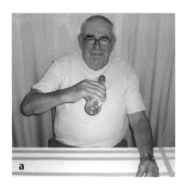 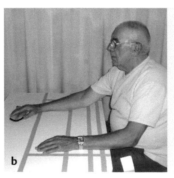

Tinetti Test				Step length and height, left free leg	
	Sitting Balance		0	L foot does not pass R foot when walking	
0	Leans or slides in chair		1	Step through R	
1	Steady, safe		0	L foot does not clear floor fully	
			1	L foot clears floor	
	Rises from chair			**Step symmetry**	
0	Unable to without help		0	Right and left step length not equal	
1	Able, uses arms to help				
2	Able without use of arms		1	Right and left step length appear equal	
	Attempts to rise			**Step continuity**	
0	Unable to without help		0	Stopping or discontinuity between steps	
1	Able, requires >1 attempt				
2	Able to rise, 1 attempt		1	Steps appear continuous	
	Immediate standing balance (first 5 s)			**Path**	
0	Unsteady (staggers, moves feet, trunk sway)		0	Marked deviation	
1	Steady but uses walker or other support		1	Mild/moderate deviation or uses w. aid	
2	Steady without walker or other support		2	Straight without walking aid	
	Standing balance (keeping feet close together)			**Trunk**	
0	Unsteady		0	Marked sway or uses walking aid	
1	Steady but wide stance and uses support		1	No sway but flex. knees or back or Uses arms for stability	
2	Narrow stance without support		2	No sway, flex., use of arms or w. aid	
	Nudged (three times with palm against patient's sternum)			**Walking time**	
0	Begins to fall		0	Heels apart	
1	Staggers, grabs, catches self		1	Heels almost touching while walking	
2	Steady				
	Eyes closed (feet are as close together as possible)			**Turning 360 degrees**	
0	Unsteady		0	Discontinuous steps	
			1	Continuous	
1	Steady		0	Unsteady (grabs, staggers)	
			1	Steady	
	Indication of gait (Immediately after told to "go")			**Sitting down**	
0	Any hesitancy or multiple attempts		0	Unsafe (misjudged distance, falls into chair)	
1	No hesitancy		1	Uses arms or not a smooth motion	
			2	Safe, smooth motion	
	Step length and height, right free leg			= Balance Score Carried Forward (maximum 16 points)	
0	R foot does not pass L foot when walking				
1	Step through L			= Gait Score (maximum 12 points)	
0	R foot does not clear floor fully			= Total Score = Balance + Gait Score (maximum 28 points)	
1	R foot clears floor				

Fig. 9.7 Tinetti Test. (Tinetti Balance Assessment Tool)

Table 9.1 Test procedures

Test	Brief description
Action Research Arm Test (ARAT)[241]	The ARAT is a motor function test to assess arm, hand, and finger activities. It tests the ability to perform unilateral arm activities and consists of 4 component tests (grasping, gripping, precision grip, gross movements) with a total of 14 test tasks to assess fine motor hand and finger functions as well as arm function. The 19 tasks are scored on a 4-level scale (0–3). The maximum possible score is 57. The test is intended to evaluate measures to improve function of the upper extremities in neurologic injuries and disorders. Required material: table and chair, blocks, sharpening stone, ball, ball bearings, marbles, glass, pipette. Required time: about 8–15 min (▶ Fig. 9.1)
Austrian Mobility Scale (AMS)[10]	This scale measures the changes in effects when mobilizing bedridden patients. As there was no overall scale for Chapter 4 "Mobility" in the category "Activity" of the International Classification of Functional Health (ICF), Ammer and coworkers developed the AMS. The practicability of the scale is verified and evaluated by simultaneously recording patient mobility according to the Rivermead Scores and the Esslinger Transfer Scale
Barthel Index[245]	The Barthel Index helps evaluate abilities with respect to activities of daily life and systematically record independence or the need for care, respectively (▶ Table 9.2)
Berg Balance Scale (BBS)[25]	The BBS was developed to measure balance and the risk of falling in geriatric medicine. Later, it was also applied to poststroke, multiple sclerosis, and brain injury patients. The BBS is regarded in physical therapy as the gold standard for measuring balance and estimating the risk of a fall. Stability and balance reaction (primarily when standing) are tested in 14 tasks on a scale from 0–4. Allowance is made for assistance. The required time is 15–20 min. Required materials include only a stopwatch, a tape measure, and a step or low stool (▶ Table 9.3)
Box and Block Test (BBT)[69]	The BBT is a motor function test to assess gross manual dexterity. The task involves moving as many blocks as possible (2.5 cm edge length) from one side of the box to the other within 60 s. The number of blocks is counted. The BBT is suitable for patients of all age levels. For patients with minimal hand and arm function, there is a floor effect (▶ Fig. 9.2)
Dynamic Gait Index (DGI)[368]	The DGI measures the patient's ability to adapt gait to different requirements of daily life (▶ Fig. 9.3)
Expanded Disability Status Scale (EDSS)[218]	The EDSS evaluates neurologic deficits in MS patients and determines the degree of severity of MS. The EDSS is too rough to describe progress in rehabilitation (▶ Table 9.4)
Freezing of Gait Questionnaire (FOGQ)[144]	Questionnaire about freezing of gait in patients with Parkinson's disease. The questionnaire consists of 6 questions that the patient answers (▶ Table 9.5)
Fugl–Meyer Test (FM)[140]	The Fugl–Meyer test can be used to measure recovery from motor problems in poststroke patients. It is divided into upper and lower extremity sections. The test is time consuming and is limited to the functional level
Functional Ambulation Categories (FAC)	Evaluation of walking ability. It is very easy to perform but has a very rough classification. This classification describes relevant "milestones" of mobility (▶ Table 9.6)
Functional Independence Measure (FIM) (Granger et al[151])	The FIM can be used with any patients who require assessment of their activities of daily life. Testing covers 18 activities of daily life. Thirteen of these items are described as motor items. They include 4 subscales: self-care, continence, transfers, and locomotion. The last 5 items are used to estimate cognitive performance. These consist of the 2 subscales communication and cognition. The individual items are scored on a scale of 1–7, where 7 indicates completely independent performance of a task within an appropriate period of time. A score of 1 indicates complete lack of independence (The patient's participation in performing the task is less than 25%). What the patient actually does in daily life is evaluated, not what he is theoretically capable of doing (▶ Table 9.7)
Functional Reach Test (FRT)[102]	The FRT is a motor function test to assess balance. It measures the patient's ability to reach forward over the length of the outstretched arms without losing balance. The patient stands next to a wall, facing parallel it. A horizontal scale is hung on the wall at shoulder height. The patient is instructed to make a fist and bend forward with outstretched arms as far as possible without losing balance. The average of 3 results out of 5 attempts is noted (▶ Fig. 9.4)

Table 9.1 Test procedures (continued)

Test	Brief description
Glasgow Coma Scale (GCS)[399]	The GCS has become a standard clinical test, although this scale is often criticized for not testing things such as light and pupil reflexes. Upon verbal instruction or stimulus, the following items are evaluated: • The best verbal response • The best motor response • Eye opening Every item is evaluated on a scale of 1–5 points. The severity of craniocerebral trauma is assigned a point value by definition: • Severe craniocerebral trauma, 3–8 points • Moderately severe craniocerebral trauma, 9–12 points • Slight craniocerebral trauma, 13–15 points
Gross Motor Function Classification System (GMFCS)	The GMFCS is a standardized, validated, and reliable system for classifying patients with infantile cerebral palsy (ICP) according to their motor impairment on a 5-point ordinal scale. The GMFCS originated from the GMFM and takes into account the motor milestones of child development
Medical Research Council Scale (MRC)	The severity of a paresis is measured with the MRC scale. In neurology, one should have the tests performed isometrically from a reflex-inhibiting initial position (▶ Table 5.4)
Würzburg Fatigue Inventory for MS (WEIMuS)	Test to document fatigue in patients with multiple sclerosis. The patient answers all the questions on a scale of 0–4 (▶ Table 9.8)
Nine Hole Peg Test (NHPT, fine motor control)[254]	The NHPT is suitable for measuring finger dexterity. The test requires only a little material and time. The NHPT measures the time the patient requires to place 9 wooden pegs 32 mm in length (9 mm in diameter) in the holes of a wooden board and then remove them again. The dominant hand is always tested first. Healthy subjects require about 30 seconds to perform the test (▶ Fig. 9.5)
Unified Parkinson's Disease Rating Scale (UPDRS)[57]	The UPDRS was published in 1987 and unified all previous scales of cardinal motor symptoms of Parkinson's disease. The UPDRS is established worldwide and can be used across the entire clinical spectrum. It covers practically all the motor symptoms and motor complications. The drawback of the UPDRS is that a few instructions with respect to evaluating individual items are not clearly defined; there is some vagueness in the text definitions of the individual degrees of severity. Because of a floor effect, it is hard to use the UPDRS to evaluate patients with mild symptoms in the early phase of Parkinson's disease. For this reason, the Movement Disorder Society developed a new version of the UPDRS, the MSD-UPDR.318
Rivermead ADL scale	The Rivermead ADL scale is usually used by occupational therapists. It measures independence in self-care (16 tasks) and in the extended household setting (15 tasks), including grocery shopping, making beds, etc
Rivermead Mobility Index	The index measures the patient's mobility on the basis of 15 tasks (from turning in bed to walking)
Stroke Impact Scale (SIS)	The SIS measures the quality of life, specifically for poststroke patients. By repeatedly querying the patient, the therapist can assess the effect of the intervention on the patient's quality of life (▶ Table 9.9)[101]
Time Walking Test	This test measures walking ability in various diseases.[253] It includes walking speed and walking endurance at different distances and times (speed at 5, 10, and 20 meters and endurance at 2, 6, and 20 minutes). The 10 meter walking test (speed) and the 6 minute test (endurance) are often used. Reference values for healthy subjects for the 6 minute test are about 600 meters for men and 500 meters for women. Reference values for the 6 minute test can be calculated as follows according to Troosters et al[407]: Walking distance(m) = 218.0 + (5.14 × height – 5.32 × age) (1.8 × weight + 51.31 × sex) (height in cm, age in years, weight in kg, and sex: 0 for men and 1 for women)[354]

Table 9.1 Test procedures (continued)

Test	Brief description
Timed "Up and Go" (TUG)[317]	The patient sits relaxed on a chair with armrests, stands up, and walks 3 meters, turns around, and goes back to the chair. The time the patient requires to return to the initial position is measured. The seat of the chair has a height of about 46 cm. The TUG is used for patients with limited ability to maintain balance. The evaluation is divided into 3 categories: less than 20 seconds, 20–30 seconds, and over 30 seconds.
Performance Oriented Mobility Assessment (POMA) or Tinetti Score[404]	The POMA measures the risk of falling in elderly persons but can also be used with other patients who have an increased risk of falling (▶Fig. 9.7)
Wolf Motor Function Test (WMFT)	The WMFT is a standardized motion test for motor function in the arm. It was originally developed for patients participating in forced-use therapy after having suffered a stroke or craniocerebral trauma. The patients perform 16 movements used in daily life (gross and fine motor skills). The quality of the movement (scale of 0–5), functionality (scale of 0–5), and the time required are evaluated (▶Fig. 9.6)

Table 9.2 Barthel Index

Activities of daily life (ADL)	Evaluation
Defecation	0 = Incontinent 1 = Occasional "accidents" (once a week) 2 = Continent
Bladder	0 = Incontinent or catheterized and not able to regulate it alone 1 = Occasional "accidents" (< once in 24 hours) 2 = Continent
Grooming	0 = Needs assistance in grooming 1 = Independent; face, hair, teeth, shaving (with appropriate aids)
Toilet use	0 = Dependent 0 = Needs some assistance, can usually do it alone 2 = Independent (sitting down, standing up, wiping, getting dressed)
Eating	0 = Not possible 1 = Needs help cutting, spreading butter, etc 2 = Independent
Transfer (bed to chair and back)	0 = Not possible, no balance when sitting 1 = A lot of help (One or two people with exertion) 2 = A little help (verbal or physical) 3 = Independent
Mobility	0 = Immobile 1 = Wheelchair 2 = Walks with the help of another person (verbal or physical) 3 = Independent (possibly with walking aids)
Getting dressed	0 = Dependent 1 = Half by themselves, half with help 2 = Independent (including buttons, zipper, belts, etc)
Stairs	0 = Not possible 2 = Needs help (verbal, physical, or aids) 2 = Independent
Bathing	0 = Dependent 1 = Independent (includes showering)
Total	0–20 points

Table 9.3 Berg Balance Scale (BBS)

Items of the Berg Balance Scale	1	2	3	4
From sitting to standing	☐	☐	☐	☐
Standing upright without support	☐	☐	☐	☐
Sitting upright without support with the feet on the floor	☐	☐	☐	☐
From standing to sitting	☐	☐	☐	☐
Transfers	☐	☐	☐	☐
Standing with eyes closed	☐	☐	☐	☐
Standing upright with the feet together	☐	☐	☐	☐
Leaning forward with the arms raised	☐	☐	☐	☐
Picking something up off the floor	☐	☐	☐	☐
Turning around and looking back over the left or right shoulder	☐	☐	☐	☐
Turning in place (360 degrees)	☐	☐	☐	☐
Dynamically shifting weight while upright without support. How often can the foot touch the footstool?	☐	☐	☐	☐
Staying upright without support with one foot in front of the other	☐	☐	☐	☐
Standing upright on one leg	☐	☐	☐	☐

Note: Maximum score: 56; less than 36 points indicates a likely fall.

Table 9.4 Expanded Disability Status Scale (EDSS)

Grade	
0.0	Normal neurologic examination (grade 0 in all functional systems)
1.0	No disability, minimal abnormality in one functional system, i. e., grade 1)
1.5	No disability, minimal abnormality in more than one functional system (except for cerebral function; more than one grade 1)
2.0	Minimal disability in one functional system (one system: grade 2, others: 0 or 1)
2.5	Minimal disability in two functional systems (two systems: grade 2, others: 0 or 1)
3.0	Moderate disability in one functional system (one system: grade 3, another: 0 or 1) or slight disability in 3 or 4 functional systems (3 or 4 systems: grade 2, others: 0 or 1)
3.5	Fully able to walk but with moderate disability in one functional system (grade 3) and one or two systems (grade 2), or two systems (grade 3), or five systems (grade 2, others: 0 or 1)
4.0	Able to walk without assistance and rest for at least 500 meters, active for about 12 hours per day despite relatively severe disability (one functional system: grade 4, others: 0 or 1)
4.5	Able to walk without assistance and rest for about 200 meters, able to work the entire day, certain restrictions in activity, requires minimal help, relatively severe disability (one functional system: grade 4, others: 0 or 1)
5.0	Able to walk without assistance and rest for about 200 meters; disability is severe enough to impair daily activities (such as working the entire day without special measures; one functional system: grade 5, others: 0 or 1, or combinations of lower grades that exceed the specifications of level 4)
5.5	Able to walk without assistance and rest for about 100 meters; disability is severe enough to render normal daily work impossible (FS equivalent as in level 5)
6.0	Requires intermittent support or constant support on one side (forearm crutch, cane, or splint) to walk about 100 meters without rest (FS equivalent: combination of more than two systems grade 3 plus)
6.5	Requires constant support (forearm crutch, cane, or splint) to walk about 20 meters without rest (FS equivalent as in 6.0)

Table 9.4 Expanded Disability Status Scale (EDSS) (continued)

Grade	
7.0	Unable, even with assistance, to walk more than 5 meters, largely confined to a wheelchair and transfers self without help (FS equivalent: combination of more than two systems: grade 4 plus, rarely pyramidal tract: grade 5 alone)
7.5	Unable to walk more than a few steps; confined to a wheelchair, requires help for transfer, moves wheelchair alone but cannot spend the whole day in the wheelchair; may require a motorized wheelchair (FS equivalent as for 7)
8.0	Largely confined to bed or wheelchair; grooms self largely independently, usually with good use of the arms (FS equivalent: combination of usually grade 4 plus in multiple systems)
8.5	Largely confined to bed even during the day; good use of the arms occasionally, can groom self occasionally (FS equivalent as for 8)
9.0	Helpless patient in bed; can eat and communicate (FS equivalent is a combination, usually grade 4 plus)
9.5	Completely helpless patient unable to eat, swallow, or communicate (FS equivalent is a combination, almost exclusively grade 4 plus)
10.0	Death due to multiple sclerosis

Abbreviation: FS = functional system.

Table 9.5 Freezing of Gait Questionnaire (FOGQ), German version.

In your worst condition, do you walk?	
Normally	☐
Nearly normally	☐
A little more slowly	☐
Slowly but completely independently	☐
With support or a walking aid	☐
Not at all because I am unable to walk	☐
Does your gait disturbance affect your daily life and your independence?	
Not at all	☐
Only slightly	☐
Moderately	☐
Severely	☐
I am unable to lead an independent life	☐
Do you have the feeling that your feet stick to the ground (freeze) when you walk, turn, or try to start walking?	
Never	☐
Very rarely, about once a month	☐
Rarely, about once a week	☐
Often, about once a day	☐
Constantly, whenever I walk	☐
How long did your longest freezing episode last?	
Never occurred	☐
1–2 seconds	☐
3–10 seconds	☐
11–30 seconds	☐
Unable to walk for over 30 seconds	☐

Table 9.5 Freezing of Gait Questionnaire (FOGQ), German version. (continued)

How long does your hesitation typically last when you start to walk?	
No hesitation	☐
Longer than 1 second	☐
Longer than 3 seconds	☐
Longer than 10 seconds	☐
Longer than 30 seconds	☐
How long does your hesitation typically last when you turn (freezing while turning)?	
No hesitation	
Continue turning within 12 seconds	
Continue turning within 3–10 seconds	
Continue turning within 11–30 seconds	
Unable to continue turning after more than 30 seconds	

Table 9.6 Functional Ambulation Categories (FAC)

Walking ability	FAC values
The patient cannot walk or needs the assistance of two or more therapists when walking	0
The patient is dependent on constant help from another person who helps bear weight and maintain balance	1
The patient is dependent on constant or intermittent help from another person to maintain balance and coordination	2
The patient is dependent on verbal support from or the accompaniment of another person, whereas immediate physical assistance is excluded	3
The patient walks independently on a level surface and requires only slight assistance in cases such as climbing stairs or when on difficult surfaces	4
The patient is able to walk independently in every respect	5

Source: Mehrholz, J. Den Gang zuverlässig beurteilen. pt_Zeitschrift für Physiotherapeuten. 2007;(11)1096–1104

Table 9.7 Functional Independence Measure (FIM)

Functional Independence Measure (FIM)	1	2	3	4	5	6	7
Self-care							
A Eating and drinking	☐	☐	☐	☐	☐	☐	☐
B Grooming	☐	☐	☐	☐	☐	☐	☐
C Bathing, showering, washing	☐	☐	☐	☐	☐	☐	☐
D Dressing upper body	☐	☐	☐	☐	☐	☐	☐
E Dressing lower body	☐	☐	☐	☐	☐	☐	☐
F Personal hygiene	☐	☐	☐	☐	☐	☐	☐
Continence							
G Bladder control	☐	☐	☐	☐	☐	☐	☐
H Bowel control	☐	☐	☐	☐	☐	☐	☐

Table 9.7 Functional Independence Measure (FIM) (continued)

Functional Independence Measure (FIM)	1	2	3	4	5	6	7
Transfers							
I Chair, bed, wheelchair	☐	☐	☐	☐	☐	☐	☐
J Toilet seat	☐	☐	☐	☐	☐	☐	☐
K Shower, bathtub	☐	☐	☐	☐	☐	☐	☐
Locomotion							
L Walking, wheelchair*	☐	☐	☐	☐	☐	☐	☐
M Climbing stairs	☐	☐	☐	☐	☐	☐	☐
Communication							
N Comprehension acoustic, visual*	☐	☐	☐	☐	☐	☐	☐
O Expression verbal, nonverbal	☐	☐	☐	☐	☐	☐	☐
Cognitive skills							
P Social behavior	☐	☐	☐	☐	☐	☐	☐
Q Problem solving	☐	☐	☐	☐	☐	☐	☐
R Memory	☐	☐	☐	☐	☐	☐	☐

1 = completely dependent, <25%
2 = completely dependent, 25–49%
3 = partially dependent, 40–74%
4 = partially dependent, 75–99%
5 = partially dependent with supervision
6 = limited independence
7 = complete independence
*Please delete if not applicable.

Table 9.8 Würzburg Fatigue Inventory for multiple sclerosis (WEIMuS)

	During the last week	0	1	2	3	4
1	Fatigue was one of the three symptoms that impaired me the most					
2	I was unable to think clearly because of my fatigue					
3	Because of my fatigue, I had difficulty keeping my thoughts together at home or at work					
4	Fatigue impaired physical activity					
5	Because of my fatigue, I had difficulty concentrating					
6	Physical activity led to increased fatigue					
7	Because of my fatigue, I was forgetful					
8	Fatigue prevented me from performing certain tasks and duties					
9	Because of my fatigue, I had difficulty completing things that required me to concentrate					
10	Because of my fatigue, I had little motivation to do things that required me to concentrate					
11	Fatigue influenced my work, family, or social life					
12	Fatigue caused frequent problems for me					
13	Because of my fatigue, I was not very attentive					
14	Because of my fatigue, my thinking was slower					
15	Because of my fatigue, I had difficulty following things for an extended period of time					
16	Fatigue influenced my exercise tolerance					

Note: Every statement is evaluated on a scale of 0 (never) to 4 (almost always).

Table 9.9 Excerpts for the Stroke Impact Scale

Questions about strength				
In the past week, how much strength do you think you had				
a: in the arm that was more severely affected by the stroke?				
A lot of strength ⑤	A good amount of strength ④	Some strength ③	Little strength ②	No strength at all ①
b: when grasping with the hand that was more severely affected by the stroke?				
A lot of strength ⑤	A good amount of strength ④	Some strength ③	Little strength ②	No strength at all ①

Questions about emotions				
In the past week, how often				
a: were you sad?				
Never ⑤	Rarely ④	Occasionally ③	Usually ②	Always ①
b: did you have the feeling that there is no one close to you?				
Never ⑤	Rarely ④	Occasionally ③	Usually ②	Always ①
c: did you have the feeling of being a burden to others?				
Never ⑤	Rarely ④	Occasionally ③	Usually ②	Always ①

Questions about activities of daily life				
In the past 2 weeks, how difficult was it for you				
a: to cut your food with a knife and fork?				
Not difficult at all ⑤	A little difficult ④	Rather difficult ③	Very difficult ②	Not possible ①
b: to dress your upper body (from the waist up)?				
Not difficult at all ⑤	A little difficult ④	Rather difficult ③	Very difficult ②	Not possible ①

Note: Questionnaire about the impact of a stroke.

10 Further Reading

[1] Ackermann H. Ataxie. Assessment und Management. In: Frommelt P, Lösslein H, eds. NeuroRehabilitation. 3. Aufl. Heidelberg: Springer; 2010

[2] Ada L, Canning CG, Low SL. Stroke patients have selective muscle weakness in shortened range. Brain. 2003; 126(Pt 3):724–731

[3] Agre JC, Rodriquez AA, Franke TM, Swiggum ER, Harmon RL, Curt JT. Low-intensity, alternate-day exercise improves muscle performance without apparent adverse effect in postpolio patients. Am J Phys Med Rehabil. 1996; 75(1):50–58

[4] Agre JC, Rodriquez AA, Franke TM. Strength, endurance, and work capacity after muscle strengthening exercise in postpolio subjects. Arch Phys Med Rehabil. 1997; 78(7):681–686

[5] Aitkens SG, McCrory MA, Kilmer DD, Bernauer EM. Moderate resistance exercise program: its effect in slowly progressive neuromuscular disease. Arch Phys Med Rehabil. 1993; 74(7):711–715

[6] Alacamlioglu Y, Amann-Griober H, Prager C. Schlaganfallrehabilitation – Teil 2. Österr Z. Phys Med Rehabil. 2002; 12(1):3–8

[7] Alexanderson H. Exercise: an important component of treatment in the idiopathic inflammatory myopathies. Curr Rheumatol Rep. 2005; 7(2):115–124

[8] Alexanderson H, Lundberg IE. The role of exercise in the rehabilitation of idiopathic inflammatory myopathies. Curr Opin Rheumatol. 2005; 17(2):164–171

[9] Altschuler EL, Wisdom SB, Stone L, et al. Rehabilitation of hemiparesis after stroke with a mirror. Lancet. 1999; 353(9169):2035–2036

[10] Ammer K, Bochdansky T, Prager Ch. Patientenmobilisierung und Mobilitätsskala. Österr Z Phys Med Rehabil. 2004; 14(1):29–34

[11] Andersen LL, Zeeman P, Jørgensen JR, et al. Effects of intensive physical rehabilitation on neuromuscular adaptations in adults with poststroke hemiparesis. J Strength Cond Res. 2011; 25(10):2808–2817

[12] Ansved T. Muscle training in muscular dystrophies. Acta Physiol Scand. 2001; 171(3):359–366

[13] Archer T, Fredriksson A, Johansson B. Exercise alleviates Parkinsonism: clinical and laboratory evidence. Acta Neurol Scand. 2011; 123(2):73–84

[14] Arya KN, Pandian S, Verma R, Garg RK. Movement therapy induced neural reorganization and motor recovery in stroke: a review. J Bodyw Mov Ther. 2011; 15(4):528–537

[15] AWMF online. www.awmf.org/leitlinien/detail/ll/024–018.html-Schädel-Hirn-Trauma im Kindesalter; Stand: 05.10.2012

[16] Balducci S, Iacobellis G, Parisi L, et al. Exercise training can modify the natural history of diabetic peripheral neuropathy. J Diabetes Complications. 2006; 20(4):216–223

[17] Banaschewski T, Besmens F, Zieger H, Rothenberger A. Evaluation of sensorimotor training in children with ADHD. Percept Mot Skills. 2001; 92(1):137–149

[18] Bardt T. Multimodales zerebrales Monitoring bei Patienten mit schwerem Schädel-Hirn-Trauma [Dissertation]. Berlin: Medizinische Fakultät der Charité; 2001

[19] Barnes MP, Ward AB. Textbook of rehabilitation. Oxford: Oxford University Press; 2000

[20] Bauer HL, Kesserling J, Beer S. Medizinische Rehabilitation und Nachsorge bei Multipler Sklerose. Stuttgart: G. Fischer; 1989

[21] Bazelier MT, de Vries F, Bentzen J, et al. Incidence of fractures in patients with multiple sclerosis: the Danish National Health Registers. Mult Scler. 2012; 18(5):622–627

[22] Beer S, Kesselring J. Neurorehabilitation bei multipler Sklerose. Schweiz Arch Neurol Psychiatr. 2009; 2:46–51

[23] Elbert T, Rockstroh B, Bulach D, Meinzer M, Taub E. Die Fortentwicklung der Neurorehabilitation auf verhaltensneurowissenschaftlicher Grundlage. Beispiel constraint-induced-therapie. Nervenarzt. 2003; 74(4):334–342

[24] Bello-Haas VD, Florence JM, Kloos AD, et al. A randomized controlled trial of resistance exercise in individuals with ALS. Neurology. 2007; 68(23):2003–2007

[25] Berg K, Wood-Dauphinee S, Williams JI, , Gayton, D. Clinical and laboratory measures of postural balance in an elderly population. Physiother Can. 1989; 41:304–311

[26] Berlit P. Klinische Neurologie. 3. Aufl. Heidelberg: Springer; 2011

[27] Bernier JN, Perrin DH. Effect of coordination training on proprioception of the functionally unstable ankle. J Orthop Sports Phys Ther. 1998; 27(4):264–275

[28] Bernsen RA, de Jager AE, van der Meché FG, Suurmeijer TP. How Guillain-Barre patients experience their functioning after 1 year. Acta Neurol Scand. 2005; 112(1):51–56

[29] Berschin G, Schmiedeberg I, Sommer HM. Zum Einsatz von Vibrationskrafttraining als spezifisches Schnellkrafttrainingsmittel in Sportspielen. Leistungssport. 2003; 33(4):11–13

[30] Bethesda, MD. National Institutes of Health (US). Plasticity and Learning:2007

[31] Hitec. Bizeps, Trizeps & Co. Available at:www.3sat.de/page/?source=/hitec/144776/index.html (Erstsendung 31.05.2010). Stand: 03.05.2012

[32] Bjarnadottir OH, Konradsdottir AD, Reynisdottir K, Olafsson E. Multiple sclerosis and brief moderate exercise. A randomised study. Mult Scler. 2007; 13(6):776–782

[33] Blair SN, Kohl HW, Gordon NF, Paffenbarger RS, Jr. How much physical activity is good for health? Annu Rev Public Health. 1992; 13:99–126

[34] BMBF. http://www.gesundheitsforschung-bmbf.de/de/4494. Stand: 10.08.2013

[35] Böhme P, Arnold CR. Muskeldystrophie vom Gliedergürteltyp – Therapieergebnisse physikalischer Behandlungen unter stationären Bedingungen. Akt Neurol. 2004; 31:1–5

[36] Borg G. Anstrengungsempfinden und körperliche Aktivität. Dtsch Arztebl. 2004; 101:1016–1021

[37]   Borg G. Physical performance and perceived exertion. Studia Psychologia et Paedagogica. Series altera. Investigationes XI. Lund: Gleerup; 1962

[38]   Borggraefe I, Meyer-Heim A, Kumar A, Schaefer JS, Berweck S, Heinen F. Improved gait parameters after robotic-assisted locomotor treadmill therapy in a 6-year-old child with cerebral palsy. Mov Disord. 2008; 23(2):280–283

[39]   Borggräfe I, Kumar A, Schäfer JS, et al. Robotergestützte Laufbandtherapie für Kinder mit zentralen Gangstörungen. Monatsschr Kinderheilkd. 2007; 155(6):529–534

[40]   Bosco C, Iacovelli M, Tsarpela O, et al. Hormonal responses to whole-body vibration in men. Eur J Appl Physiol. 2000; 81(6):449–454

[41]   Bosco C. The influence of whole body vibration on jumping performance. Biol Sport. 1998; 15(3):157–164

[42]   Bös K, Brehm W. Gesundheitssport – Abgrenzungen und Ziele. dvs-Informationen. 1999; 14(2)–9–18

[43]   Bös K. Motorische Leistungsfähigkeit von Kindern und Jugendlichen. In: Schmidt W, Hartmann-Tews I, Brettschneider WD (Hrsg). Erster Deutscher Kinder- und Jugendsportbericht. Schorndorf: Karl Hoffmann; 2003;85–107

[44]   Braumann KM, Stiller N. Bewegungstherapie bei Internistischen Erkrankungen. Heidelberg: Springer; 2010

[45]   Brodal P. The Central Nervous System: Structure and Function. Oxford: Oxford University Press; 1995

[46]   Bruyere O, Wuidart MA, Di Palma E, et al. Controlled whole body vibration to decrease fall risk and improve health-related quality of life of nursing home residents. Arch Phys Med Rehabil. 2005; 86(2):303–307

[47]   Burkhardt A. Vibrationstraining in der Physiotherapie – Wippen mit Wirkung. Physiopraxis. 2006; 9:22–25

[48]   Buschfort R, Hess A, Breit M, et al. Gruppentherapie im Armlabor für den schwer und mäßig betroffenen Arm nach Schlaganfall: Akzeptanz, Auslastung und erste klinische Ergebnisse. Neuro Rehabil. 2009; 15(6):337–343

[49]   Bütefisch C, Hummelsheim H, Denzler P, Mauritz KH. Repetitive training of isolated movements improves the outcome of motor rehabilitation of the centrally paretic hand. J Neurol Sci. 1995; 130(1):59–68

[50]   Buttler DS. Mobilisation des Nervensystems. 2. korr. Nachdr. Heidelberg:Springer; 1998

[51]   Canning CG, Ada L, Adams R, O'Dwyer NJ. Loss of strength contributes more to physical disability after stroke than loss of dexterity. Clin Rehabil. 2004; 18(3):300–308

[52]   Cano-de-la-Cuerda R, Pérez-de-Heredia M, Miangolarra-Page JC, Muñoz-Hellín E, Fernández-de-Las-Peñas C. Is there muscular weakness in Parkinson's disease? Am J Phys Med Rehabil. 2010; 89(1):70–76

[53]   Cardinale M, Lim J. Electromyography activity of vastus lateralis muscle during whole-body vibrations of different frequencies. J Strength Cond Res. 2003; 17(3):621–624

[54]   Carr JH, Shepherd RB. Stroke rehabilitation. Guidelines for exercise and training to optimize motor skill. Oxford: Butterworth Heinemann; 2003

[55]   Carter GT. Rehabilitation Management of Neuromuscular Disease. 2006. http://emedicine.medscape.com. Accessed on January 26, 2012

[56]   Ceballos-Baumann A. Relevante Studien zur Parkinson-Therapie 2009–2010. Medikamente, aktivierende Therapien und tiefe Hirnstimulation. Nervenheilkunde. 2010; 29:825–833

[57]   Ceballos-Baumann A, Ebersbach G. Aktivierende Therapien bei Parkinson-Syndromen. Stuttgart: Thieme; 2008

[58]   Ceballos-Baumann A, Conrad B. Bewegungsstörungen. 2. Aufl. Stuttgart: Thieme; 2005

[59]   Chan KM, Amirjani N, Sumrain M, Clarke A, Strohschein FJ. Randomized controlled trial of strength training in post-polio patients. Muscle Nerve. 2003; 27(3):332–338

[60]   Charité. Bed Rest Studie. www.esa.int/esaCP/SEM4E-JXJD1E_Germany_0.html; http://www.charite.de/zmk/bedrest/pdf_doc/PM-WeltRaum-Medizin.pdf; Berlin

[61]   Chase RA, Cullen JK, Jr, Sullivan SA, Ommaya AK. Modification of intention tremor in man. Nature. 1965; 206(983):485–487

[62]   Cherng RJ, Liu CF, Lau TW, Hong RB. Effect of treadmill training with body weight support on gait and gross motor function in children with spastic cerebral palsy. Am J Phys Med Rehabil. 2007; 86(7):548–555

[63]   Chetlin RD, Gutmann L, Tarnopolsky M, Ullrich IH, Yeater RA. Resistance training effectiveness in patients with Charcot-Marie-Tooth disease: recommendations for exercise prescription. Arch Phys Med Rehabil. 2004; 85(8):1217–1223

[64]   Chi L, Masani K, Miyatani M, et al. Cardiovascular response to functional electrical stimulation and dynamic tilt table therapy to improve orthostatic tolerance. J Electromyogr Kinesiol. 2008; 18(6):900–907

[65]   Choi JT, Bastian AJ. Adaptation reveals independent control networks for human walking. Nat Neurosci. 2007; 10(8):1055–1062

[66]   Colombo G, Joerg M, Schreier R, Dietz V. Treadmill training of paraplegic patients using a robotic orthosis. J Rehabil Res Dev. 2000; 37(6):693–700

[67]   Cooper AR, Page AS, Foster LJ, Qahwaji D. Commuting to school: are children who walk more physically active? Am J Prev Med. 2003; 25(4):273–276

[68]   Crizzle AM, Newhouse IJ. Is physical exercise beneficial for persons with Parkinson's disease? Clin J Sport Med. 2006; 16(5):422–425

[69]   Cromwell FS. Occupational therapists manual for basic skills assessment:primary prevocational evaluation. Pasadena: Fair Oaks Printing; 1965

[70]   Cup EH, Pieterse AJ, Ten Broek-Pastoor JM, et al. Exercise therapy and other types of physical therapy for patients with neuromuscular diseases: a systematic review. Arch Phys Med Rehabil. 2007; 88(11):1452–1464

[71]   Bello-Haas VD, Florence JM, Kloos AD, et al. A randomized controlled trial of resistance exercise in individuals with ALS. Neurology. 2007; 68(23):2003–2007

[72]   Dalgas U, et al. Krafttraining bei schubförmig verlaufender Multipler Sklerose. Akt Neurol. 2010; 37:213–218

[73]   Dalgas U, Ingemann-Hansen T, Stenager E. Physical exercise and MS – recommendations. Int MS J. 2009; 16(1):5–11

[74]   Dalgas U, Kant M, Stenager E. Resistance training in relapsing-remitting Multiple Sclerosis. Act Neurol. 2010; 37(5):213–218

[75] Damiano DL. Activity, activity, activity: rethinking our physical therapy approach to cerebral palsy. Phys Ther. 2006; 86(11):1534–1540

[76] Damiano DL, Abel MF. Functional outcomes of strength training in spastic cerebral palsy. Arch Phys Med Rehabil. 1998; 79(2):119–125

[77] Dawes H, Korpershoek N, Freebody J, et al. A pilot randomised controlled trial of a home-based exercise programme aimed at improving endurance and function in adults with neuromuscular disorders. J Neurol Neurosurg Psychiatry. 2006; 77(8):959–962

[78] de Souza-Teixeira F, Costilla S, Ayán C, García-López D, González-Gallego J, de Paz JA. Effects of resistance training in multiple sclerosis. Int J Sports Med. 2009; 30(4):245–250

[79] Delecluse C, Roelants M, Verschueren S. Strength increase after whole-body vibration compared with resistance training. Med Sci Sports Exerc. 2003; 35(6):1033–1041

[80] Dengler R. Eine Broschüre der Deutschen Gesellschaft für Muskelkranke DGM e.V. 2002

[81] Dettmers Ch, Bülau P, Weiller C, eds. Rehabilitaion der Multiplen Sklerose. Bad Honnef: Hippocampus; 2010

[82] Dettmers Ch, Stephan KM. Motorische Therapie nach Schlaganfall. Bad Honnef:Hippocampus; 2011

[83] Dettmers C, Sulzmann M, Ruchay-Plössl A, Gütler R, Vieten M. Endurance exercise improves walking distance in MS patients with fatigue. Acta Neurol Scand. 2009; 120(4):251–257

[84] Dettmers C, Teske U, Hamzei F, Uswatte G, Taub E, Weiller C. Distributed form of constraint-induced movement therapy improves functional outcome and quality of life after stroke. Arch Phys Med Rehabil. 2005; 86(2):204–209

[85] Deuschl G, Eggert K, Oertel WH, et al. Parkinson-Krankheit. In: Oertel WH, Deuschl G, Poewe W, Hrsg. Parkinsonsyndrom und andere Bewegungsstörungen. Stuttgart: Thieme; 2012

[86] Deutsche Gesellschaft für Neurologie,Hrsg. Akuttherapie des ischämischen Schlaganfalls: Leitlinien der Deutschen Gesellschaft für Neurologie. 2009

[87] Di Fabio RP, Soderberg J, Choi T, Hansen CR, Schapiro RT. Extended outpatient rehabilitation: its influence on symptom frequency, fatigue, and functional status for persons with progressive multiple sclerosis. Arch Phys Med Rehabil. 1998; 79(2):141–146

[88] Diemer F, Sutor V. Praxis der medizinischen Trainingstherapie. 2. Aufl. Stuttgart: Thieme; 2011

[89] Diener HC, Putzki N, eds. Leitlinien für Diagnostik und Therapie in der Neurologie. 4. Aufl. Stuttgart: Thieme; 2008

[90] Dietz V. Hintergrund: Central Pattern Generator – Hypothesen und Evidenz. Neuroreha. 2010; 2(1):28–32

[91] Dietz V. Spinal cord pattern generators for locomotion. Clin Neurophysiol. 2003; 114(8):1379–1389

[92] Dietz V, Berger W. Neue Aspekte zur Pathophysiologie der Spastik. Nervenarzt. 1987; 58(7):399–402

[93] Dietz V, Müller R. Degradation of neuronal function following a spinal cord injury:mechanisms and countermeasures. Brain. 2004; 127(Pt 10):2221–2231

[94] Dimitrijevic MR, Gerasimenko Y, Pinter MM. Evidence for a spinal central pattern generator in humans. Ann N Y Acad Sci. 1998; 860:360–376

[95] Dobke B, Schüle K, Diehl W, et al. Apparativ-assistive Bewegungstherapie in der Schlaganfallrehabilitation. Neurol Rehabil. 2010; 16(4):173–185

[96] Dobkin BH. Clinical practice. Rehabilitation after stroke. N Engl J Med. 2005; 352(16):1677–1684

[97] Dodd KJ, Taylor NF, Shields N, Prasad D, McDonald E, Gillon A. Progressive resistance training did not improve walking but can improve muscle performance, quality of life and fatigue in adults with multiple sclerosis: a randomized controlled trial. Mult Scler. 2011; 17(11):1362–1374

[98] Dromerick AW. Evidence-based rehabilitation: the case for and against constraint-induced movement therapy. J Rehabil Res Dev. 2003; 40(1):vii–ix

[99] Drory VE, Goltsman E, Reznik JG, Mosek A, Korczyn AD. The value of muscle exercise in patients with amyotrophic lateral sclerosis. J Neurol Sci. 2001; 191(1)(2):133–137

[100] Duncan PW. Synthesis of intervention trials to improve motor recovery following stroke. Top Stroke Rehabil. 1997; 3(4):1–20

[101] Duncan PW, Wallace D, Lai SM, Johnson D, Embretson S, Laster LJ. The stroke impact scale version 2.0. Evaluation of reliability, validity, and sensitivity to change. Stroke. 1999; 30(10):2131–2140

[102] Duncan PW, Weiner DK, Chandler J, Studenski S. Functional reach: a new clinical measure of balance. J Gerontol. 1990; 45(6):M192–M197

[103] Ebersbach G, Ceballos-Baumann A. Aktivierende therapien bei parkinson-syndromen. Nervenheilkunde. 2008; 8:746–756

[104] Ebersbach G, Ebersbach A, Edler D, et al. Comparing exercise in Parkinson's disease–the Berlin LSVT®BIG study. Mov Disord. 2010; 25(12):1902–1908

[105] Ebersbach G, Wissel J. Parkinsonkrankheit und Dystonie. In: Frommelt P, Lösslein H, Hrsg. NeuroRehabilitation. 3. Aufl. Heidelberg: Springer; 2010

[106] Edwards S. Longer term management for patients with residual or progressive disability. In: Edwards S, Hrsg. Neurological Physiotherapy. 2. Aufl. London:Churchill Livingstone; 2002:255–273

[107] Eek MN, Tranberg R, Zügner R, Alkema K, Beckung E. Muscle strength training to improve gait function in children with cerebral palsy. Dev Med Child Neurol. 2008; 50(10):759–764

[108] Eickhof C. Wiederherstellung der Innervationsfähigkeit für Zielmotorik durch ein systematisches repetitives Basistraining. In: Eickhof C, Hrsg. Grundlage der Therapie bei erworbenen Lähmungen. München: Plaum Verlag; 2001

[109] Einarsson G. Muscle conditioning in late poliomyelitis. Arch Phys Med Rehabil. 1991; 72(1):11–14

[110] Einspieler C, Marschik PB. Central Pattern Generators und ihre Bedeutung für die fötale Motorik. Klin Neurophysiol. 2012; 43(1):16–21

[111] Elbert T, Pantev C, Wienbruch C, Rockstroh B, Taub E. Increased cortical representation of the fingers of the left hand in string players. Science. 1995; 270(5234):305–307

[112] Elbert T, Rockstroh B, Bulach D, Meinzer M, Taub E. Die Fortentwicklung der Neurorehabilitation auf verhaltensneurowissenschaftlicher Grundlage. Beispiel Constraint-induced-Therapie. Nervenarzt. 2003; 74(4):334–342

[113] Enoka RM. Neuromechanics of human movement. 4th ed. Champaign, IL: Human Kinetic; 2008

[114] Ettema GJC. Contractile behavior in skeletal muscle-tendon unit during small amplitude sine wave perturbations. J Biomech. 1996; 9:1147–1155

[115] Farbu E, Gilhus NE, Barnes MP, et al. EFNS guideline on diagnosis and management of post-polio syndrome. Report of an EFNS task force. Eur J Neurol. 2006; 13(8):795–801

[116] Farley BG, Koshland GF. Training BIG to move faster: the application of the speed-amplitude relation as a rehabilitation strategy for people with Parkinson's disease. Exp Brain Res. 2005; 167(3):462–467

[117] Fasoli SE, Trombly CA, Tickle-Degnen L, Verfaellie MH. Effect of instructions on functional reach in persons with and without cerebrovascular accident. Am J Occup Ther. 2002; 56(4):380–390

[118] Fheodoroff K. Prädiktoren von ADL in der neurologischen Rehabilitation. In:Österreichische Gesellschaft für Neurologie, Hrsg. Neurologisch. Fachmagazin für Neurologie. Wien: Medmedia-Verlag; 2008:S15–S18

[119] Filipi ML, Kucera DL, Filipi EO, Ridpath AC, Leuschen MP. Improvement in strength following resistance training in MS patients despite varied disability levels. NeuroRehabilitation. 2011; 28(4):373–382

[120] Fischer CP. Interleukin-6 in acute exercise and training: what is the biological relevance? Exerc Immunol Rev. 2006; 12:6–33

[121] Fisher MA, Langbein WE, Collins EG, Williams K, Corzine L. Physiological improvement with moderate exercise in type II diabetic neuropathy. Electromyogr Clin Neurophysiol. 2007; 47(1):23–28

[122] Fitts PM, Posner MI. Human Performance. Oxford: Brooks and Cole; 1967

[123] Flansbjer UB, Lexell J, Brogårdh C. Long-term benefits of progressive resistance training in chronic stroke: a 4-year follow-up. J Rehabil Med. 2012; 44(3):218–221

[124] Flansbjer UB, Miller M, Downham D, Lexell J. Progressive resistance training after stroke: effects on muscle strength, muscle tone, gait performance and perceived participation. J Rehabil Med. 2008; 40(1):42–48

[125] Foerster O. Kompensatorische Übungstherapie. In: Vogt H, Hrsg. Handbuch der Therapie der Nervenkrankheiten. Jena: Gustav Fischer; 1916

[126] Foerster O. Übungstherapie. In: Bumke O, Foerster O, Hrsg. Handbuch der Neurologie, Bd 8. Berlin: Springer; 1936

[127] Forssberg H. Ontogeny of human locomotor control. I. Infant stepping, supported locomotion and transition to independent locomotion. Exp Brain Res. 1985; 57(3):480–493

[128] Freivogel S, Schmalohr D, Mehrholz J. Improved walking ability and reduced therapeutic stress with an electromechanical gait device. J Rehabil Med. 2009; 41(9):734–739

[129] Freivogel S. Forced-use-Therapie. In: Mehrholz J, Hrsg. Neuroreha nach Schlaganfall. Stuttgart: Thieme; 2011

[130] Freivogel S. Motorische Rehabilitation nach Schädelhirntrauma. München: Pflaum Verlag; 1997

[131] Freivogel S, Hummelsheim H. Qualitätskriterien und Leitlinien für die motorische Rehabilitation von Patienten mit Hemiparesen. Aktuelle Neurol. 2003; 30:401–406

[132] Frenkel HS. Die Behandlung der Tabische Ataxie mit Hilfe der Übung:Compensatorische Uebungstherapie, ihre Grundlagen und Technik. Leipzig: F. C. W. Vogel; 1900

[133] Frevel D, Mäurer M. Sport bei Multipler Sklerose. Akt Neurol. 2012; 39:248–253

[134] Friedmann B. Neuere Entwicklungen im Krafttraining. Muskuläre Anpassungsreaktionen bei verschiedenen Krafttrainingsmethoden. Dtsch Z Sportmed. 2007; 58(1):12–18

[135] Fries W, Freivogel S. Motorische Rehabilitation. In: Frommelt P, Lössein H, Hrsg. NeuroRehabilitation. 3. Aufl. Heidelberg: Springer; 2010

[136] Fries W, Freivogel S, Beck B. Rehabilitation von Störungen der Willkürmotorik. In: Frommelt P, Grötzbach H, Hrsg. Neurorehabilitation. Berlin: Blackwell Wissenschaftsverlag; 1999

[137] Fries W, Lössl H, Wagenhäuser S. Teilhaben! – Neue Konzepte der Neuro-Rehabilitation – für eine erfolgreiche Rückkehr in Alltag und Beruf. Stuttgart: Thieme; 2007

[138] Frommelt P. Historische Perspektive der Neurorehabilitation. In: Frommelt P, Lösslein H, Hrsg. NeuroRehabilitation. 3. Aufl. Heidelberg: Springer 2010

[139] Frommelt P, Lösslein H. NeuroRehabilitation. 3. Aufl. Heidelberg: Springer; 2010

[140] Fugl-Meyer AR, Jääskö L, Leyman I, Olsson S, Steglind S. The post-stroke hemiplegic patient. A method for evaluation of physical performance. Scand J Rehabil Med. 1975; 7(1):13–31

[141] Ganten D, Spahl T, Deichmann T. Die Steinzeit steckt uns in den Knochen:Gesundheit als Erbe der Evolution. München u. Zürich: Piper; 2011

[142] Garssen MP, Bussmann JB, Schmitz PI, et al. Physical training and fatigue, fitness, and quality of life in Guillain-Barré syndrome and CIDP. Neurology. 2004; 63(12):2393–2395

[143] Gehlsen GM, Grigsby SA, Winant DM. Effects of an aquatic fitness program on the muscular strength and endurance of patients with multiple sclerosis. Phys Ther. 1984; 64(5):653–657

[144] Giladi N, Shabtai H, Simon ES, Biran S, Tal J, Korczyn AD. Construction of freezing of gait questionnaire for patients with Parkinsonism. Parkinsonism Relat Disord. 2000; 6(3):165–170

[145] Gleyse J. Gymnastik als Gestaltung des Körpers in der Frühen Neuzeit: Diskurse, Praktiken oder Transgressionen. In: von Mallinckrodt R, Hg. Bewegtes Leben. Körpertechniken in der Frühen Neuzeit. Wiesbaden: Harrassowitz Verlag; 2008:125–142

[146] Globas C, Macko RF, Luft AR. Role of walking-exercise therapy after stroke. Expert Rev Cardiovasc Ther. 2009; 7(8):905–910

[147] Goodwin VA, Richards SH, Taylor RS, Taylor AH, Campbell JL. The effectiveness of exercise interventions for people with Parkinson's disease: a systematic review and meta-analysis. Mov Disord. 2008; 23(5):631–640

[148] Gordon AM, Charles J, Wolf SL. Methods of constraint-induced movement therapy for children with hemiplegic cerebral palsy: development of a child-friendly intervention for improving upper-extremity function. Arch Phys Med Rehabil. 2005; 86(4):837–844

[149] Gorter H, Holty L, Rameckers EE, Elvers HJ, Oostendorp RA. Changes in endurance and walking ability through

functional physical training in children with cerebral palsy. Pediatr Phys Ther. 2009; 21(1):31–37

[150] Granacher, et al. Sensomotorisches Training in der Bewegungstherapie, der Verletzungsprophylaxe und im Sport. Medizinische Orthopädieschuhtechnik –Sonderheft Sensomotorik 2006:72–79

[151] Granger CV, Hamilton BB, Keith RA, et al. Advances in functional assessment for medical rehabilitation. Top Geriatr Rehabil. 1986; 1:59–74

[152] Gresham GE, Kelly-Hayes M, Wolf PA, Beiser AS, Kase CS, D'Agostino RB. Survival and functional status 20 or more years after first stroke: the Framingham Study. Stroke. 1998; 29(4):793–797

[153] Gruber M, Gollhofer A. Impact of sensorimotor training on the rate of force development and neural activation. Eur J Appl Physiol. 2004; 92(1)(2):98–105

[154] Gutenbrunner Ch, Weimann G. Krankengymnastische Methoden und Konzepte. Heidelberg: Springer 2004

[155] Haas CT. Vibrationstraining, Biomechanische Stimulation und Stochastische Resonanz-Therapie: pt_Zeitschrift für Physiotherapeuten. 2008; 60:728–744

[156] Haas CT, Schmidtbleicher D. Zu den Effekten mechanischer Schwingungsreize bei Morbus Parkinson. Rheuma Aktuell. 2002; 3:8–10

[157] Haas CT, Turbanski S, Kessler K, Schmidtbleicher D. The effects of random whole-body-vibration on motor symptoms in Parkinson's disease. NeuroRehabilitation. 2006; 21(1):29–36

[158] Haber P, Tomasitis J. Medizinische Trainingstherapie – Anleitung für die Praxis. Heidelberg: Springer; 2006

[159] Halle M, Schmidt-Trucksäss A, Hambrecht R, et al. Sporttherapie in der Medizin–Evidenzbasierte Prävention und Therapie. Stuttgart: Schattauer; 2008

[160] Hamzei F. Update Physiotherapie. Evidenzbasierte NeuroReha. Stuttgart: Thieme; 2008

[161] Hamzei F, Krüger H, Peters M, et al. Shaping-induced movement therapy for lower extremity (SIMT) – a pilot study. Neurol Rehabil. 2012; 18(4):236–241

[162] Handschin C, Spiegelman BM. The role of exercise and PGC1α in inflammation and chronic disease. Nature. 2008; 454(7203):463–469

[163] Hanisch F, Zierz S. Metabolische und toxische Myopathien. ÄP Neurologie Psychiat 2011;2

[164] Harris JE, Eng JJ. Strength training improves upper-limb function in individuals with stroke:a meta-analysis. Stroke. 2010; 41(1):136–140

[165] Haskell WL, Lee IM, Pate RR, et al; American College of Sports Medicine. American Heart Association. Physical activity and public health: updated recommendation for adults from the American College of Sports Medicine and the American Heart Association. Circulation. 2007; 116(9):1081–1093

[166] Hauptmann B. Grundzüge der Rehabilitation von Muskelerkrankungen. In:Hummelsheim H, Hrsg. Neurologische Rehabilitation. Heidelberg: Springer; 1998

[167] Heilmittelkatalog. Ludwigsburg: InteliMed. GmbH Verlag; 2011

[168] Heitkamp HC, Horstmann T, Mayer F, Weller J, Dickhuth HH. Gain in strength and muscular balance after balance training. Int J Sports Med. 2001; 22(4):285–290

[169] Henze T. Symptomatische Therapie der Multiplen Sklerose. Stuttgart: Thieme; 2005

[170] Herman T, Giladi N, Hausdorff JM. Treadmill training for the treatment of gait disturbances in people withParkinson's disease: a mini-review. J Neural Transm (Vienna). 2009; 116(3):307–318

[171] Hermsdörfer J. Handfunktionsstörungen: Assessment und Management. In: Frommelt P, Lösslein H, Hrsg. NeuroRehabilitation. 3. Aufl. Heidelberg: Springer; 2010

[172] Hesse S, Bertelt C, Jahnke MT, et al. Treadmill training with partial body weight support compared with physiotherapy in nonambulatory hemiparetic patients. Stroke. 1995; 26(6):976–981

[173] Hesse S, Bertelt C, Schaffrin A, Malezic M, Mauritz KH. Restoration of gait in nonambulatory hemiparetic patients by treadmill training with partial body-weight support. Arch Phys Med Rehabil. 1994; 75(10):1087–1093

[174] Hesse S, Schulte-Tigges G, Konrad M, Bardeleben A, Werner C. Robot-assisted arm trainer for the passive and active practice of bilateral forearm and wrist movements in hemiparetic subjects. Arch Phys Med Rehabil. 2003; 84(6):915–920

[175] Hesse S, Tomelleri C, Bardeleben A, Werner C, Waldner A. Robot-assisted practice of gait and stair climbing in nonambulatory stroke patients. J Rehabil Res Dev. 2012; 49(4):613–622

[176] Hesse S, Waldner A, Tomelleri C. Innovative gait robot for the repetitive practice of floor walking and stair climbing up and down in stroke patients. J Neuroeng Rehabil. 2010; 7:30–40

[177] Hesse S, Werner C. Automatisierte motorische Rehabilitation. In: Frommelt P, Lösslein H, Hrsg. NeuroRehabilitation. 3. Aufl. Heidelberg: Springer; 2010

[178] Hesse S, Werner C, Brocke J. Maschinen- und Robotereinsatz in der Neurorehabilitation. Orthopädie-Technik. 2009; 2:74–77

[179] Hinderer SR, Gupta S. Functional outcome measures to assess interventions for spasticity. Arch Phys Med Rehabil. 1996; 77(10):1083–1089

[180] Hirsch MA, Toole T, Maitland CG, Rider RA. The effects of balance training and high-intensity resistance training on persons with idiopathic Parkinson's disease. Arch Phys Med Rehabil. 2003; 84(8):1109–1117

[181] Hoehn MM, Yahr MD. Parkinsonism: onset, progression and mortality. Neurology. 1967; 17(5):427–442

[182] Hogan N, Krebs HI, Charnarong J, Sharon A. Interactive robotics therapist. US Patent No. 5466213. Cambridge: Massachusetts Institute of Technology; 1995

[183] Hohlfeld R, Melms A, Schneider C, et al. Therapy of myasthenia gravis and myasthenic syndromes. In: Brandt T, Caplan LR, Dichgans J, Diener HC, Kennard C, eds. Neurological disorders – course and treatment. Amsterdam: Elsevier; 2003:1341–1362

[184] Hollmann W, Hettinger T. Sportmedizin. 3. Aufl. Stuttgart: Schattauer; 1990

[185] Hollmann W. Geleitwort. In: Halle M, Schmidt-Trucksäss A, Hambrecht R, Berg A, Hrsg. Sporttherapie in der Medizin – evidenzbasierte Prävention und Therapie. Stuttgart: Schattauer; 2008

[186] Holmes G. The cerebellum of man. Brain. 1939; 62:1–30

[187] Hömberg V, Boering D, Krause H, et al. Modulares Stufenkonzept für die Behandlung motorischer Störungen. In: Dettmers Ch, Stephan KM, Hrsg. Motorische Therapie nach Schlaganfall. Bad Honnef: Hippocampus Verlag, 2011

[188] Hoppeler H, Baum O, Mueller M, et al. Molekulare Mechanismen der Anpassungsfähigkeit der Skelettmuskulatur.

Schweizerische Zeitschrift für Sportmedizin und Sporttraumatologie. 2011; 59(1):6–13

[189] Hotz M, Mewes J, Biniek R. Komaassoziierte Neuropathie. Nervenarzt. 1997; 68(8):659–663

[190] Huber M. Das Richtige üben. Transfer motorischer Fertigkeiten. Physiopraxis. 2008; 4:28–31

[191] Hufschmidt A, Mauritz KH. Chronic transformation of muscle in spasticity: a peripheral contribution to increased tone. J Neurol Neurosurg Psychiatry. 1985; 48(7):676–685

[192] Hummelsheim H. Rehabilitation bei zentralen Paresen. Schweiz Arch Neurol Psychiatr. 2009; 160(7):299–301

[193] Hummelsheim H. Neurologische Rehabilitation. Heidelberg: Springer; 1998

[194] Hund E. Critical illness – Polyneuropathie und –myopathie. Intensivmed Notfallmed. 2003; 40(3):203–211

[195] Hüter-Becker A, Dölken M. Biomechanik, Bewegungslehre, Leistungsphysiologie, Trainingslehre. Stuttgart: Thieme; 2005

[196] Ivey FM, Macko RF, Ryan AS, Hafer-Macko CE. Cardiovascular health and fitness after stroke. Top Stroke Rehabil. 2005; 12(1):1–16

[197] Jackson JH. On the anatomical and physiological localisation of movement in the brain. In: Taylor J, ed. Selected writings of John Hughlings Jackson. New York; 1958

[198] Jeschke D, Zeilberger K. Altern und körperliche Aktivität. Dtsch Arztebl. 2004; 101:789–798

[199] Jöbges M, Heuschkel G, Pretzel C, Illhardt C, Renner C, Hummelsheim H. Repetitive training of compensatory steps: a therapeutic approach for postural instability in Parkinson's disease. J Neurol Neurosurg Psychiatry. 2004; 75(12):1682–1687

[200] Jones DR, Speier J, Canine K, Owen R, Stull GA. Cardiorespiratory responses to aerobic training by patients with postpoliomyelitis sequelae. JAMA. 1989; 261(22):3255–3258

[201] Kampfl A, Schmutzhard E, Franz G, et al. Prediction of recovery from post-traumatic vegetative state with cerebral magnetic-resonance imaging. Lancet. 1998; 351(9118):1763–1767

[202] Kelm J, Ahlhelm F, Regitz T, Pape D, Schmitt E. Kontrolliertes dynamisches Krafttraining bei Patienten mit neuromuskulären Erkrankungen. Fortschr Neurol Psychiatr. 2001; 69(8):359–366

[203] Kern C. Klettern mit Multiple Sklerose: Therapieoption oder nur ein Traum? e&l. 2010; 5:27–31

[204] Kerschan-Schindl K, Grampp S, Henk C, et al. Wholebody vibration exercise leads to alterations in muscle blood volume. Clin Physiol. 2001; 21(3):377–382

[205] Kidd G, Lawes N, Musa I. Understanding Neuromuscular Plasticity: A Basis for Clinical Rehabilitation. London: Edward Arnold; 1992

[206] Kileff J, Ashburn A. A pilot study of the effect of aerobic exercise on people with moderate disability multiple sclerosis. Clin Rehabil. 2005; 19(2):165–169

[207] Kilmer DD, McCrory MA, Wright NC, Aitkens SG, Bernauer EM. The effect of a high resistance exercise program in slowly progressive neuromuscular disease. Arch Phys Med Rehabil. 1994; 75(5):560–563

[208] King MB, Tinetti ME. Falls in community-dwelling older persons. J Am Geriatr Soc. 1995; 43(10):1146–1154

[209] Kleinöder H. Safety consideration in vibration training. Book of Abstracts. 8th annual congress European College of Sports Science. Salzburg; 2003

[210] Knecht S, Hesse S, Oster P. Rehabilitation after stroke. Dtsch Arztebl Int. 2011; 108(36):600–606

[211] Koch JW. Medizinische Trainingstherapie bei neuromuskulären Erkrankungen. 2009. www.muskelgesellschaft.ch/downloads/medizin/K_Koch_Trainingstherapie_25.1.2011.pdf Accessed: December 17, 2012

[212] Koch JW, Burgunder JM. Rehabilitation bei neuromuskulären Erkrankungen: Stellenwert der medizinischen Trainingstherapie. Schweiz Arch Neurol Psychiatr. 2002; 153:69–81

[213] Kollen BJ, Lennon S, Lyons B, et al. The effectiveness of the Bobath concept in stroke rehabilitation: what is the evidence? Stroke. 2009; 40(4):e89–e97

[214] Koller W, Kase S. Muscle strength testing in Parkinson's disease. Eur Neurol. 1986; 25(2):130–133

[215] Kramer A, Dettmers C, Gruber M. Gleichgewichtstraining in der neurologischen Rehabilitation. Neurologie und Rehabilitation. 2013; 1:27–33

[216] Kramers-de Quervain IA, Stüssi E, Stacoff A. Ganganalyse beim Gehen und Laufen. Schweizerische Zeitschrift für Sportmedizin und Sporttraumatologie. 2008; 56(2):35–42

[217] Kriz JL, Jones DR, Speier JL, Canine JK, Owen RR, Serfass RC. Cardiorespiratory responses to upper extremity aerobic training by postpolio subjects. Arch Phys Med Rehabil. 1992; 73(1):49–54

[218] Kurtzke JF. Rating neurologic impairment in multiple sclerosis: an expanded disability status scale (EDSS). Neurology. 1983; 33(11):1444–1452

[219] Kuys SS, Brauer SG, Ada L. Higher-intensity treadmill walking during rehabilitation after stroke is feasible and not detrimental to walking pattern or quality: a pilot randomized trial. Clin Rehabil. 2010; 4:10

[220] Kwakkel G, Wagenaar RC, Koelman TW, Lankhorst GJ, Koetsier JC. Effects of intensity of rehabilitation after stroke. A research synthesis. Stroke. 1997; 28(8):1550–1556

[221] Lajoie Y, Teasdale N, Bard C, Fleury M. Attentional demands for static and dynamic equilibrium. Exp Brain Res. 1993; 97(1):139–144

[222] Lamontagne A, Fung J. Faster is better: implications for speed-intensive gait training after stroke. Stroke. 2004; 35(11):2543–2548

[223] Lamprecht S. NeuroReha bei Multipler Sklerose – Physiotherapie – Sport–Selbsthilfe. Stuttgart: Thieme; 2008

[224] Lance JW. Pathophysiology of spasticity and clinical experience with Baclofen. In: Feldman RG, Young RR, Koella WP, eds. Spasticity: Disordered Motor Control. Chicago: Year Book Medical Publishers; 1980:185–203

[225] Landesmann E. Die Therapie an den Wiener Kliniken – Ein Verzeichnis der wichtigsten, an denselben gebräuchlichen Heilmethoden und Recepte. Leipzig u. Wien: Frank Deutikel; 1888

[226] Latash ML, Anson JG. What are "normal movements" in atypical populations? Behav Brain Sci. 1996; 19(1):55–68

[227] Laufens G, Poltz W, Prinz E, et al. Verbesserung der Lokomotion durch kombinierte Laufband-/Vojta-Physiotherapie bei ausgewählten MS-Patienten. Phys Med Rehab Kuror. 1999; 9:187–189

[228] Laupheimer M, Härtel S, Schmidt S, et al. Forced Exercise – Auswirkungen eines MOTOmed®-Trainings auf

parkinsontypische motorische Dysfunktionen. Neurol Rehabil. 2011; 17(5/6):239–246

[229] Lazik D. Klettern mit Patienten nach Schlaganfall. Physiopraxis. 2007; 5(3):32–35

[230] Lehmann-Horn F, Lerche H, Mitrovic N, Jurkat-Rott K. Ionenkanalerkrankungen – Krankheitsbilder. Dtsch Arztebl. 2000; 97(27):A-1902–A-1907

[231] Lerche H, Mitrovic N, Jurkat-Rott K, et al. Ionenkanalerkrankungen, allgemeine Charakteristika und Pathomechanismen. Dtsch Arztebl. 2000; 97(26):A-1826–A-1831

[232] Lernier-Frankiel M, Vargas S, Brown M, et al. Functional community ambulation: what are your criteria? Clinical Management in Physical Therapy. 1986; 6(2):12–15

[233] Leven KH, ed. Antike Medizin – ein Lexikon. München: C.H. Beck; 2005

[234] Lexell J, Flansbjer UB. Muscle strength training, gait performance and physiotherapy after stroke. Minerva Med. 2008; 99(4):353–368

[235] Liebisch U. Kortikale Verarbeitung von bewegungs- und sprachrelevanten visuellen Stimuli bei Gehörlosen, Gebärdensprachdolmetschern und Hörenden: Eine Untersuchung mit funktioneller Kernspintomografie [Dissertation]. Halle:Martin-Luther-Universität Halle-Wittenberg; 2005

[236] Liepert J. Evidenzbasierte Verfahren in der motorischen Rehabilitation. J Neurol Neurochir Psychiatr. 2010; 11:5–10

[237] Lindeman E, Spaans F, Reulen J, Leffers, P, Drukker, J. Progressive resistance training in neuromuscular patients. Effects on force and surface EMG. J Electromyogr Kinesiol. 1999; 9(6):379–384

[238] Lindeman E, Leffers P, Spaans F, et al. Strength training in patients with myotonic dystrophy and hereditary motor and sensory neuropathy: a randomized clinical trial. Arch Phys Med Rehabil. 1995; 76(7):612–620

[239] Lo AC, Guarino PD, Richards LG, et al. Robot-assisted therapy for long-term upper-limb impairment after stroke. N Engl J Med. 2010; 362(19):1772–1783

[240] Lum PS, Burgar CG, Van der Loos M, Shor PC, Majmundar M, Yap R. MIME robotic device for upper- limb neurorehabilitation in subacute stroke subjects: A follow-up study. J Rehabil Res Dev. 2006; 43(5): 631–642

[241] Lyle RC. A performance test for assessment of upper limb function in physical rehabilitation treatment and research. Int J Rehabil Res. 1981; 4(4):483–492

[242] MacKay-Lyons M. Central pattern generation of locomotion: a review of the evidence. Phys Ther. 2002; 82(1):69–83

[243] Mackett R, et al. The health benefits of walking to School. Paper for the Sustrans national conference. Leicester; 2003

[244] Macko RF, Ivey FM, Forrester LW, et al. Treadmill exercise rehabilitation improves ambulatory function and cardiovascular fitness in patients with chronic stroke: a randomized, controlled trial. Stroke. 2005; 36(10):2206–2211

[245] Mahoney FI, Barthel DW. Functional evaluation: the Barthel Index. Md State Med J. 1965; 14:61–65

[246] Majsak MJ. Application of motor learning principles to the stroke population. Top Stroke Rehabil. 1996; 3(2):37–59

[247] Malfait N, Shiller DM, Ostry DJ. Transfer of motor learning across arm configurations. J Neurosci. 2002; 22(22):9656–9660

[248] Malin JP, Sindern E. Das akute Guillain-Barré-Syndrom. Dtsch Arztebl. 1996; 93:A-1895–A-1898

[249] Marchese R, Diverio M, Zucchi F, Lentino C, Abbruzzese G. The role of sensory cues in the rehabilitation of parkinsonian patients: a comparison of two physical therapy protocols. Mov Disord. 2000; 15(5):879–883

[250] Marder E, Bucher D. Central pattern generators and the control of rhythmic movements. Curr Biol. 2001; 11(23):R986–R996

[251] Marschall F, Kolb C, Wittstadt T, Meyer, T. Zum Verhältnis von metabolischer und kardialer Beanspruchung auf drei unterschiedlichen Ergometertypen: Fahrrad, Cross-Trainer und Stairmaster. Dtsch Z Sportmed. 2006; 10:255–259

[252] Masson F, Thicoipe M, Aye P, et al; Aquitaine Group for Severe Brain Injuries Study. Epidemiology of severe brain injuries: a prospective population-based study. J Trauma. 2001; 51(3):481–489

[253] Masur H. Skalen und Scores in der Neurologie. Stuttgart: Thieme; 2000

[254] Mathiowetz V, Weber K, Kashman N, G, Volland, et al. Adult norms for Nine Hole Peg test of finger dexterity. Occup Ther J Res. 1985; 5:25–38

[255] Mattern-Baxter K. ICP Laufbandtraining. Pediatr Phys Ther. 2009; 21:12–22

[256] Mayer J, Hermann HD. Mentales Training. Grundlagen und Anwendungen in Sport, Rehabilitation, Arbeit und Wirtschaft. 2. Aufl. Heidelberg: Springer; 2011; 150–165

[257] Mayr H, Ammer K. Ganzkörpervibration (GKV) – Methoden und Indikationen. Eine Literaturübersicht. Österr Z Phys Med Rehabil. 2007; 17(1):12–22

[258] McDonald CM. Limb contractures in progressive neuromuscular disease and the role of stretching, orthotics, and surgery. Phys Med Rehabil Clin N Am. 1998; 9(1):187–211

[259] Meek C, Pollock A, Potter J, Langhorne P. A systematic review of exercise trials post stroke. Clin Rehabil. 2003; 17(1):6–13

[260] Mehrholz J. Das Tempo macht's – Geschwindigkeitstraining auf dem Laufband. Neuroreha. 2010; 1:15–19

[261] Mehrholz J. Frühphase Schlaganfall. Physiotherapie und medizinische Versorgung. Stuttgart: Thieme; 2008

[262] Mehrholz J. Kardiovaskuläres Training nach Schlaganfall. In: Dettmers Ch, Stephan KM, Hrsg. Motorische Therapie nach Schlaganfall. Bad Honnef:Hippokampus, 2011a

[263] Mehrholz J. Neuroreha nach Schlaganfall. Stuttgart: Thieme; 2011b

[264] Mehrholz J, Friis R, Kugler J, Twork S, Storch A, Pohl M. Treadmill training for patients with Parkinson's disease. Cochrane Database Syst Rev. 2010; 20(1):CD007830

[265] Mester J, Spitzenfeil P, Schwarzer J, Seifriz F. Biological reaction to vibration--implications for sport. J Sci Med Sport. 1999; 2(3):211–226

[266] Merians AS, Poizner H, Boian R, Burdea G, Adamovich S. Sensorimotor training in a virtual reality environment: does it improve functional recovery poststroke? Neurorehabil Neural Repair. 2006; 20(2):252–267

[267] Mertens HG. Die disseminierte Neuropathie nach Koma. Nervenarzt. 1963; 32:71–79

[268] Miller GJ, Light KE. Strength training in spastic hemiparesis: should it be avoided? NeuroRehabilitation. 1997; 9(1):17–28

[269] Miltner WH, Bauder H, Sommer M, Dettmers C, Taub E. Effects of constraint-induced movement therapy on patients with chronic motor deficits after stroke: a replication. Stroke. 1999; 30(3):586–592

[270] Miyai I, Fujimoto Y, Ueda Y, et al. Treadmill training with body weight support: its effect on Parkinson's disease. Arch Phys Med Rehabil. 2000; 81(7):849–852

[271] Möllmann FT. Epidemiologie, Unfallursachen und akutklinische Initialversorgung beim Schädel-Hirn-Trauma [Dissertation]. Münster: Westfälische Wilhelms-Universität; 2006

[272] Morgan MH. Ataxia--its causes, measurement, and management. Int Rehabil Med. 1980; 2(3):126–132

[273] Morris ME, Martin CL, Schenkman ML. Striding out with Parkinson disease: evidence-based physical therapy for gait disorders. Phys Ther. 2010; 90(2):280–288

[274] Mostert S, Kesselring J. Effects of a short-term exercise training program on aerobic fitness, fatigue, health perception and activity level of subjects with multiple sclerosis. Mult Scler. 2002; 8(2):161–168

[275] Motl RW, McAuley E, Snook EM, Gliottoni RC. Physical activity and quality of life in multiple sclerosis: intermediary roles of disability, fatigue, mood, pain, self-efficacy and social support. Psychol Health Med. 2009; 14(1):111–124

[276] Mulcare JA. Multiple sclerosis. In: American College of Sports Medicine's. Exercise management for persons with chronic diseases and disabilities. Champaign, Illinois: Human Kinetics; 1997

[277] Mulder T. Das adaptive Gehirn. Stuttgart: Thieme; 2007

[278] Müller, O, Günther, M, Krauss, I, Horstmann, T. Physical characterization of the therapeutic device Posturomed as a measuring device--presentation of a procedure to characterize balancing ability [Article in German] Biomed Tech (Berl). 2004; 49(3):56–60

[279] Nadeau S, Arsenault AB, Gravel D, Bourbonnais D. Analysis of the clinical factors determining natural and maximal gait speeds in adults with a stroke. Am J Phys Med Rehabil. 1999; 78(2):123–130

[280] Nelles G, Hesse S, Hummelsheim H. Motorische Rehabilitation nach Schlaganfall. In: Diener, HC, Hacke W, Hrsg. Leitlinien für Diagnostik und Therapie in der Neurologie. Stuttgart: Thieme; 2002:237–242

[281] Neupert M, Hamzei F. Kann Kinesio-Tape die Schmerzen nach einer durch Schlaganfall bedingten Hemiparese induzierte Schultersubluxation verbessern? Neurol Rehabil. 2012; 18(2):95–98

[282] Nogaki H, Fukusako T, Sasabe F, Negoro K, Morimatsu M. Muscle strength in early Parkinson's disease. Mov Disord. 1995; 10(2):225–226

[283] Nollet F, Beelen A, Sargeant AJ, de Visser M, Lankhorst GJ, de Jong BA. Submaximal exercise capacity and maximal power output in polio subjects. Arch Phys Med Rehabil. 2001; 82(12):1678–1685

[284] O'Dwyer NJ, Ada L, Neilson PD. Spasticity and muscle contracture following stroke. Brain. 1996; 119(Pt 5):1737–1749

[285] Oesch P, Hilfiker R, Keller S, et al. Assessment in der muskuloskelettalen Rehabilitation. Bern: Huber; 2007

[286] Oken BS, Kishiyama S, Zajdel D, et al. Randomized controlled trial of yoga and exercise in multiple sclerosis. Neurology. 2004; 62(11):2058–2064

[287] Ortner K, Pott C. Mobil im Alltag. Stolpersteine überwinden. In: Fries W, Lössl H, Wagenhäuser S, Hrsg. Teilhaben! Stuttgart: Thieme; 2007

[288] Osten P. Die Modellanstalt. Über den Aufbau einer „modernen Krüppelfürsorge, 1905-1933. Frankfurt: Mabuse; 2004

[289] Oujamaa L, Relave I, Froger J, Mottet D, Pelissier JY. Rehabilitation of arm function after stroke. Literature review. Ann Phys Rehabil Med. 2009; 52(3):269–293

[290] Paffenbarger RS, Jr, Hyde RT, Wing AL, Lee IM, Jung DL, Kampert JB. The association of changes in physical-activity level and other lifestyle characteristics with mortality among men. N Engl J Med. 1993; 328(8):538–545

[291] Page SJ, Levine P, Sisto S, Johnston MV. A randomized efficacy and feasibility study of imagery in acute stroke. Clin Rehabil. 2001; 15(3):233–240

[292] Pak S, Patten C. Strengthening to promote functional recovery poststroke: an evidence-based review. Top Stroke Rehabil. 2008; 15(3):177–199

[293] Pang MYC, Eng JJ, Dawson AS, Gylfadóttir S. The use of aerobic exercise training in improving aerobic capacity in individuals with stroke: a meta-analysis. Clin Rehabil. 2006; 20(2):97–111

[294] Pate RR, Pratt M, Blair SN, et al. Physical activity and public health. A recommendation from the Centers for Disease Control and Prevention and the American College of Sports Medicine. JAMA. 1995; 273(5):402–407

[295] Paterno MV, Myer GD, Ford KR, Hewett TE. Neuromuscular training improves single-limb stability in young female athletes. J Orthop Sports Phys Ther. 2004; 34(6):305–316

[296] Patrick E, Ada L. The Tardieu Scale differentiates contracture from spasticity whereas the Ashworth Scale is confounded by it. Clin Rehabil. 2006; 20(2):173–182

[297] Patten J. Neurological differential diagnosis. 2nd ed. London:Springer;1996

[298] Pedersen BK. Exercise-induced myokines and their role in chronic diseases. Brain Behav Immun. 2011; 25(5):811–816

[299] Pendt LK, Reuter I, Müller H. Motor skill learning, retention, and control deficits in Parkinson's disease. PLoS One. 2011; 6(7):e21669

[300] Perlmutter E, Gregory PC. Rehabilitation treatment options for a patient with paraneoplastic cerebellar degeneration. Am J Phys Med Rehabil. 2003; 82(2):158–162

[301] Perry J, Garrett M, Gronley JK, Mulroy SJ. Classification of walking handicap in the stroke population. Stroke. 1995; 26(6):982–989

[302] Petajan JH, Gappmaier E, White AT, Spencer MK, Mino L, Hicks RW. Impact of aerobic training on fitness and quality of life in multiple sclerosis. Ann Neurol. 1996; 39(4):432–441

[303] Petajan JH, White AT. Recommendations for physical activity in patients with multiple sclerosis. Sports Med. 1999; 27(3):179–191

[304] Pfeiffer G. Rehabilitation neuromuskulärer Erkrankungen. In: Frommelt P, Lösslein H, Hrsg. NeuroRehabilitation. 3. Aufl. Heidelberg: Springer; 2010

[305] Pfitzner A, Flachenecker P, Zettl UK. Die Effekte von Rehabilitation und Ausdauertraining auf die Leistungsfähigkeit bei Patienten mit MS: Ergebnisse einer randomisierten prospektiven Studie. Akt Neurol. 2009; 36(Suppl 2):172

[306] Physiolexikon. Physiotherapie von A–Z. Stuttgart: Thieme; 2010

[307] Platz T. Evidenzbasierte Armrehabilitation. Eine systematische Literaturübersicht. Nervenarzt. 2003; 74(10):841–849

[308] Platz T. IOT – Impairment-Oriented Training/ Schädigungsorientiertes Training; Theorie und deutschsprachige Manuale für Therapie und Assessment. Baden-Baden:Deutscher Wissenschafts-Verlag; 2006

[309] Platz T. Schädigungsorientiertes Training in der Armrehabilitation. In: Hamzei F, Hrsg. Update Physiotherapie. Evidenzbasierte NeuroReha. Stuttgart: Thieme; 2008:101–119

[310] Platz T, Eickhof C, van Kaick S, et al. Impairment-oriented training or Bobath therapy for severe arm paresis after stroke: a single-blind, multicentre randomized controlled trial. Clin Rehabil. 2005; 19(7):714–724

[311] Platz T, Pinkowski C, van Wijck F, Kim IH, di Bella P, Johnson G. Reliability and validity of arm function assessment with standardized guidelines for the Fugl-Meyer Test, Action Research Arm Test and Box and Block Test: a multicentre study. Clin Rehabil. 2005; 19(4):404–411

[312] Platz T, Roschka S. Rehabilitative Therapie bei Armparese nach Schlaganfall. Neurol Rehabil. 2009; 15(2):81–106

[313] Platz T, van Kaick S. Motorisches Assessment bei Patienten mit Schlaganfall. In: Dettmers Ch, Bülau P, Weiller C, Hrsg. Schlaganfallrehabilitation. Bad Honnef: Hippocampus; 2007

[314] Platz T, van Kaick S, Möller L, Freund S, Winter T, Kim IH. Impairment-oriented training and adaptive motor cortex reorganisation after stroke: a fTMS study. J Neurol. 2005; 252(11):1363–1371

[315] Platz T, Winter T, Müller N, Pinkowski C, Eickhof C, Mauritz KH. Arm ability training for stroke and traumatic brain injury patients with mild arm paresis: a single-blind, randomized, controlled trial. Arch Phys Med Rehabil. 2001; 82(7):961–968

[316] Plotnik M, Dagan Y, Gurevich T, Giladi N, Hausdorff JM. Effects of cognitive function on gait and dual tasking abilities in patients with Parkinson's disease suffering from motor response fluctuations. Exp Brain Res. 2011; 208(2):169–179

[317] Podsiadlo D, Richardson S. The timed "up and go": a test of basic functional mobility for frail elderly persons. J Am Geriatr Soc. 1991; 39:142–149

[318] Poewe W, Wenning G, Bürk K. Skale zur Beurteilung von Schweregrad und Beeinträchtigung bei Bewegungsstörungen. In: Oertel WH, Deuschl G, Poewe W, Hrsg. Parkinson-Syndrome und andere Bewegungsstörungen. Stuttgart: Thieme; 2012

[319] Pohl M, Mehrholz J, Ritschel C, Rückriem S. Speed-dependent treadmill training in ambulatory hemiparetic stroke patients: a randomized controlled trial. Stroke. 2002; 33(2):553–558

[320] Pohl M, Rockstroh G, Rückriem S, Mrass G, Mehrholz J. Immediate effects of speed-dependent treadmill training on gait parameters in early Parkinson's disease. Arch Phys Med Rehabil. 2003; 84(12):1760–1766

[321] Prado-Medeiros CL, Silva MP, Lessi GC, et al. Muscle atrophy and functional deficits of knee extensors and flexors in people with chronic stroke. Phys Ther. 2012; 92(3):429–439

[322] Praet SF, Jonkers RA, Schep G, et al. Long-standing, insulin-treated type 2 diabetes patients with complications respond well to short-term resistance and interval exercise training. Eur J Endocrinol. 2008; 158(2):163–172

[323] Prinz JP. Elisée Bouny. Der Erfinder des Fahrradergometers. In: Tittel K, Arndt KH, Hollmann W, Hrsg. Sportmedizin. Gestern – heute – morgen. Leipzig:Barth; 1993:78–81

[324] Quaney BM, Boyd LA, McDowd JM, et al. Aerobic exercise improves cognition and motor function poststroke. Neurorehabil Neural Repair. 2009; 23(9):879–885

[325] Quasthoff S, Kieseier BC. Akutes Guillian-Barré-Syndrom. Management of neuromuscular diseases. Deutsche Gesellschaft für Muskelkranke e.V. München:Arcis; o.J

[326] Radlinger L, Bachmann W, Homburg J, et al. Rehabilitatives Krafttraining. Stuttgart: Thieme; 1998

[327] Raes P. Der Einfluss verschiedener Lernstrategien auf die Erfolgsrate beim motorischen Lernen [Dissertation]. Freiburg i.Br.: Albert-Ludwigs-Universität; 2012

[328] Rampello A, Franceschini M, Piepoli M, et al. Effect of aerobic training on walking capacity and maximal exercise tolerance in patients with multiple sclerosis: a randomized crossover controlled study. Phys Ther. 2007; 87(5):545–555

[329] Rehwagen G. Über die Ursprünge der Krankengymnastik [Dissertation]. Düsseldorf:Heinrich-Heine-Universität; 1970

[330] Reimers CD, Knapp G, Reimers AK B Griewing. Schlaganfälle: Einfluss körperlicher Aktivität auf die Prävalenz und die Behinderung. Akt Neurol. 2012; 39:220–235

[331] Rentsch HP, Bucher PO. ICF in der Rehabilitation. Die praktische Anwendung der internationalen Klassifikation der Funktionsfähigkeit, Behinderung und Gesundheit im Rehabilitationsalltag. Idstein: Schulz-Kirchner; 2005

[332] Reuter I, Ebersbach G. Effektivität von Sport bei M. Parkinson. Akt Neurol. 2012; 39:236–247

[333] Reuter I, Mehnert S, Leone P, Kaps M, Oechsner M, Engelhardt M. Effects of a flexibility and relaxation programme, walking, and nordic walking on Parkinson's disease. J Aging Res. 2011; 2011:232473

[334] Richardson JK, Sandman D, Vela S. A focused exercise regimen improves clinical measures of balance in patients with peripheral neuropathy. Arch Phys Med Rehabil. 2001; 82(2):205–209

[335] Rickels E. Neurotraumatologie. In: Frommelt P, Lösslein H, Hrsg. NeuroRehabilitation. 3. Aufl. Heidelberg: Springer; 2010

[336] Ridgel AL, Vitek JL, Alberts JL. Forced, not voluntary, exercise improves motor function in Parkinson's disease patients. Neurorehabil Neural Repair. 2009; 23(6):600–608

[337] Riemann BL, Lephart SM. The sensorimotor system, part I: the physiologic basis of functional joint stability. J Athl Train. 2002a; 37(1):71–79

[338] Riemann BL, Lephart SM. The sensorimotor system, part II: the role of proprioception in motor control

and functional joint stability. J Athl Train. 2002b; 37(1):80–84

[339] Ritter MA, Dittrich R, Busse O, Nabavi, DG, Ringelstein, EB. Zukünftige Versorgungskonzepte des Schlaganfalls. Akt Neurol. 2012; 39:27–32

[340] Rittweger J. Acute physiological effects of training with Galileo2000: first results. Osteoporos Int. 1998; 3:8

[341] Rittweger J, Just K, Kautzsch K, Reeg P, Felsenberg D. Treatment of chronic lower back pain with lumbar extension and whole-body vibration exercise: a randomized controlled trial. Spine. 2002; 27(17):1829–1834

[342] Ritzmann R, Gollhofer A, Kramer A. The influence of vibration type, frequency, body position and additional load on the neuromuscular activity during whole body vibration. Eur J Appl Physiol. 2013; 113(1):1–11

[343] Romberg A, Virtanen A, Ruutiainen J, et al. Effects of a 6-month exercise program on patients with multiple sclerosis:a randomized study. Neurology. 2004; 63(11):2034–2038

[344] Romberg A, Virtanen A, Ruutiainen J. Long-term exercise improves functional impairment but not quality of life in multiple sclerosis. J Neurol. 2005; 252(7):839–845

[345] Rosenzweig MR, Bennett EL. Psychobiology of plasticity: effects of training and experience on brain and behavior. Behav Brain Res. 1996; 78(1):57–65

[346] Roth EJ. Heart disease in patients with stroke: incidence, impact, and implications for rehabilitation. Part 1: classification and prevalence. Arch Phys Med Rehabil. 1993; 74(7):752–760

[347] Sale A, Berardi N, Maffei L. Enrich the environment to empower the brain. Trends Neurosci. 2009; 32(4):233–239

[348] Salem Y, Godwin EM. Effects of task-oriented training on mobility function in children with cerebral palsy. NeuroRehabilitation. 2009; 24(4):307–313

[349] Salem Y et al. Strength training increases functional ability and decreases impairment in cerebral palsy children and adolescents. 2010. Doi:10.3233/ NRE-2009-0483.

[350] Saunders DH, Greig CA, Mead GE, Young A. Physical fitness training for stroke patients. Cochrane Database Syst Rev. 2009(4):CD003316

[351] Scandalis TA, Bosak A, Berliner JC, Helman LL, Wells MR. Resistance training and gait function in patients with Parkinson's disease. Am J Phys Med Rehabil. 2001; 80(1):38–43; quiz 44–46

[352] Schwend M, Haas CT. Morbus Parkinson Teil IV. Cueing, chunking und cross-modal-interaction. Interdisziplinäre Erklärungsansätze für die Gangtherapie. Physiotherapie med 2009;5:5–10

[353] Schädler S, Kool J, Lüthi H, et al. Assessments in der Neurorehabilitation. Bern: Hans Huber; 2006

[354] Der Scheld TA. 6-Minuten-Gehtest: Ein valides und reliables Verfahren zur Trainingssteuerung und Therapieevaluation in der stationären kardiologischen Rehabilitation [Dissertation]. Köln: Sporthochschule; 2007

[355] Schindl MR, Forstner C, Kern H, Hesse S. Treadmill training with partial body weight support in nonambulatory patients with cerebral palsy. Arch Phys Med Rehabil. 2000; 81(3):301–306

[356] Bös K. Motorische Leistungsfähigkeit von Kindern und Jugendlichen. Schmidt W, Hartmann-Tews I, Brettschneider WD, Hrsg. Erster Deutscher Kinder- und Jugendsportbericht. Schorndorf: Verlag Karl Hoffmann; 2003:S85–S108

[357] Schmieder F. Bewegungstherapie und Hirntraining Gailingen: Selbstverlag; 1972

[358] Schmieder F. Heilverfahren und Rehabilitation bei Hirnverletzten. Gailingen:Selbstverlag; 1967

[359] Schmieder-Wasmuth H. Die Kliniken Schmieder. In: Götz F. Gailingen, Hrsg. Geschichte einer Hochrhein-Gemeinde. Tübingen: Gulde-Druck; 2004:639–674

[360] Schneider-Gold Ch, Toyka KV. Myasthenia gravis: Pathogenese und Immuntherapie. Dtsch Arztebl. 2007; 104(7):420–426

[361] Schöler JH. Über die Anfänge der Schwedischen Heilgymnastik in Deutschland – ein Beitrag zur Geschichte der Krankengymnastik im 19. Jahrhundert [Dissertation]. Münster: Westfälische Wilhelmsuniversität; 2005

[362] Schulz KH, Heesen C. Bewegungstherapie bei Multipler Sklerose. Neurologie u Rehabilitation. 2006; 12(4):224–231

[363] Schwender U. Der Militärchirurg Joseph Clément Tissot – ein früher Verfechter derKrankengymnastik und Bewegungstherapie. Dtsch Z Sportmed. 2008; 59(2):43–45

[364] Seidenspinner D. Trainingstherapie. Heidelberg: Springer; 2005

[365] Sharp SA, Brouwer BJ, Brouwer BJ. Isokinetic strength training of the hemiparetic knee: effects on function and spasticity. Arch Phys Med Rehabil. 1997; 78(11):1231–1236

[366] Shepard RB. Weakness in patients with stroke; implication for strength training in neurorehabilitation. Phys Ther Rev. 2000; 5:227–238

[367] Shulmam LM, Katze LI, Ivey FM, et al. Exercise and gait-related disability in Parkinson disease. In: Proceedings of the 63rd annual meeting of the American Academy of Neurology. Honolulu, April 2011

[368] Shumway-Cook A, Woollacott MH. Motor Control, Theory and Practical Applications. Baltimore: Williams and Wilkins; 1995

[369] Shumway-Cook A, Woollacott MH. Motor Control: Theory and practical applications. Philadelphia: Lippincott, Williams and Wilkins; 2001

[370] Sieb JP, Schrank B. Neuromuskuläre Erkrankungen. Stuttgart: Kohlhammer; 2009

[371] Skalsky AJ, McDonald CM. Prevention and management of limb contractures in neuromuscular diseases. Phys Med Rehabil Clin N Am. 2012; 23(3):675–687

[372] Skinner JS. Körperliche Aktivität und Gesundheit: Welche Bedeutung hat die Trainingsintensität? Dtsch Z Sportmed. 2001; 6:211–214

[373] Slonim AE, Bulone L, Goldberg T, et al. Modification of the natural history of adult-onset acid maltase deficiency by nutrition and exercise therapy. Muscle Nerve. 2007; 35(1):70–77

[374] Smith RM, Adeney-Steel M, Fulcher G, Longley WA. Symptom change with exercise is a temporary phenomenon for people with multiple sclerosis. Arch Phys Med Rehabil. 2006; 87(5):723–727

[375] Solari A, Filippini G, Gasco P, et al. Physical rehabilitation has a positive effect on disability in multiple sclerosis patients. Neurology. 1999; 52(1):57–62

[376] Spector SA, Gordon PL, Feuerstein IM, Sivakumar K, Hurley BF, Dalakas MC. Strength gains without muscle injury after strength training in patients with postpolio muscular atrophy. Muscle Nerve. 1996; 19(10):1282–1290

[377] Spitzenpfeil P, et al. Strength training with whole body vibrations: single case studies and time series analyses. Presentation 4th Annual Congress of the European College of Sport Science, Rome 1999

[378] Spring H, Dvorak J, Dvorak V, et al. Theorie und Praxis der Trainingstherapie. 3. Aufl. Stuttgart: Thieme; 2008

[379] Starrost K, Liepert J. Virtuelle Realität in der neurologischen Rehabilitation. In: Dettmers Ch, Stephan KM. Motorische Therapie nach Schlaganfall. Bad Honnef:Hippocampus; 2011

[380] States RA, Salem Y, Pappas E. Overground gait training for individuals with chronic stroke: a Cochrane systematic review. J Neurol Phys Ther. 2009; 33(4):179–186

[381] Stephan KM, Krause H, Homberg V. ICF-basierte Zieldefinition als Grundlage für eine rationale Rehasteuerung. In: Dettmers Ch, Stephan KM, Hrsg. Motorische Therapie nach Schlaganfall. Bad Honnef: Hippocampus; 2011

[382] Sterr A, Freivogel S. Intensive training in chronic upper limb hemiparesis does not increase spasticity or synergies. Neurology. 2004; 63(11):2176–2177

[383] Sterr A, Freivogel S. Motor-improvement following intensive training in low-functioning chronic hemiparesis. Neurology. 2003; 61(6):842–844

[384] Sterr A, Müller MM, Elbert T, Rockstroh B, Pantev C, Taub E. Perceptual correlates of changes in cortical representation of fingers in blind multifinger Braille readers. J Neurosci. 1998; 18(11):4417–4423

[385] Störmer S. Grundlegende Kenntnisse zu Querschnittslähmungen: Ärztliche Therapie und Diagnostik. In: Hüter-Becker A, Dölken M, Hrsg. Physiotherapie in der Neurologie. Stuttgart: Thieme; 2010:266–286

[386] Sunderland A, Tinson D, Bradley L, Hewer RL. Arm function after stroke. An evaluation of grip strength as a measure of recovery and a prognostic indicator. J Neurol Neurosurg Psychiatry. 1989; 52(11):1267–1272

[387] Sünkeler IH. Epidemiologie neurologisch bedinger Behinderungen. In: Frommelt P, Lösslein H, Hrsg. NeuroRehabilitation. 3. Aufl. Heidelberg: Springer; 2010

[388] Surakka J, Romberg A, Ruutiainen J, et al. Effects of aerobic and strength exercise on motor fatigue in men and women with multiple sclerosis: a randomized controlled trial. Clin Rehabil. 2004; 18(7):737–746

[389] Suttor M, Diemer F. Morbus Parkinson Teil III – hilft Krafttraining? Physiotherapie Med. 2009; 4:5

[390] Sveen ML, Andersen SP, Ingelsrud LH, et al. Resistance training in patients with limb-girdle and becker muscular dystrophies. Muscle Nerve. 2013; 47(2):163–169

[391] Sveen ML, Jeppesen TD, Hauerslev S, Køber L, Krag TO, Vissing J. Endurance training improves fitness and strength in patients with Becker muscular dystrophy. Brain. 2008; 131(Pt 11):2824–2831

[392] Tackmann W. Neuropathien und Myopathien. In: Frommelt P, Grötzbach H, Hrsg. NeuroRehabilitation. Berlin, Wien: Blackwell; 1999

[393] Tanaka S, Hachisuka K, Ogata H. Muscle strength of trunk flexion-extension in post-stroke hemiplegic patients. Am J Phys Med Rehabil. 1998; 77(4):288–290

[394] Taub E, Miller NE, Novack TA, et al. Technique to improve chronic motor deficit after stroke. Arch Phys Med Rehabil. 1993; 74(4):347–354

[395] Taub E, Morris DM. Constraint-induced movement therapy to enhance recovery after stroke. Curr Atheroscler Rep. 2001; 3(4):279–286

[396] Taube W, Gruber M, Gollhofer A. Spinal and supraspinal adaptations associated with balance training and their functional relevance. Acta Physiol (Oxf). 2008; 193(2):101–116

[397] Taube W. Neuronale Mechanismen der posturalen Kontrolle und der Einfluss von Gleichgewichtstraining. J Neurol Neurochir Psychiatr. 2013; 14(2):55–63

[398] Taylor NF, Dodd KJ, Prasad D, Denisenko S. Progressive resistance exercise for people with multiple sclerosis. Disabil Rehabil. 2006; 28(18):1119–1126

[399] Teasdale G, Jennett B. Assessment of coma and impaired consciousness. A practical scale. Lancet. 1974; 2(7872):81–84

[400] Teixeira-Salmela LF, Olney SJ, Nadeau S, Brouwer B. Muscle strengthening and physical conditioning to reduce impairment and disability in chronic stroke survivors. Arch Phys Med Rehabil. 1999; 80(10):1211–1218

[401] Thieme H, Bayn M, Wurg M, Zange C, Pohl M, Behrens J. Mirror therapy for patients with severe arm paresis after stroke--a randomized controlled trial. Clin Rehabil. 2013; 27(4):314–324

[402] Thoumie P, Lamotte D, Cantalloube S, Faucher M, Amarenco G. Motor determinants of gait in 100 ambulatory patients with multiple sclerosis. Mult Scler. 2005; 11(4):485–491

[403] Tiffreau V, Rapin A, Serafi R, et al. Post-polio syndrome and rehabilitation. Ann Phys Rehabil Med. 2010; 53(1):42–50

[404] Tinetti ME. Performance-oriented assessment of mobility problems in elderly patients. J Am Geriatr Soc. 1986; 34(2):119–126

[405] Tinetti ME, Williams TF, Mayewski R. Tinetti Balance Assessment Tool. Fall Risk Index for elderly patients based on number of chronic disabilities. Am J Med 1986, 3(80), 429–434. Available at:http://hdcs.fullerton.edu/csa/Research/documents/TinettiPOMA.pdf

[406] Triem S, Luft AR. Nachweis von Plastizität in der Rehabilitation. Neuro Rehabil. 2009; 15(4):171–173

[407] Troosters T, Gosselink R, Decramer M. Six minute walking distance in healthy elderly subjects. Eur Respir J. 1999; 14(2):270–274

[408] Turbanski S, Haas CT, Schmidtbleicher D, Friedrich A, Duisberg P. Effects of random whole-body vibration on postural control in Parkinson's disease. Res Sports Med. 2005; 13(3):243–256

[409] Tuttle LJ, Hastings MK, Mueller MJ. A moderate-intensity weight-bearing exercise program for a person with type 2 diabetes and peripheral neuropathy. Phys Ther. 2012; 92(1):133–141

[410] Tyson SF, Connell LA, Busse ME, Lennon S. What is Bobath? A survey of UK stroke physiotherapists' perceptions of the content of the Bobath concept to treat postural control and mobility problems after stroke. Disabil Rehabil. 2009; 31(6):448–457

[411] Uhlmann A. Wolfgang Kohlrausch (1888–1980) und die Geschichte der deutschen Sportmedizin [Dissertation]. Freiburg i.Br.: Albert-Ludwigs-Universität; 2004

[412] van de Port IG, Wood-Dauphinee S, Lindeman E, Kwakkel G. Effects of exercise training programs on walking competency after stroke:a systematic review. Am J Phys Med Rehabil. 2007; 86(11):935–951

[413] van de Port IG, Kwakkel G, van Wijk I, Lindeman E. Susceptibility to deterioration of mobility long-term after stroke: a prospective cohort study. Stroke. 2006; 37(1):167–171

[414] van den Berg M, Dawes H, Wade DT, et al. Treadmill training for individuals with multiple sclerosis: a pilot randomised trial. J Neurol Neurosurg Psychiatry. 2006; 77(4):531–533

[415] van den Brand R, Heutschi J, Barraud Q, et al. Restoring voluntary control of locomotion after paralyzing spinal cord injury. Science. 2012; 336(6085):1182–1185

[416] van Nes IJ, Latour H, Schils F, Meijer R, van Kuijk A, Geurts AC. Long-term effects of 6-week whole-body vibration on balance recovery and activities of daily living in the postacute phase of stroke: a randomized, controlled trial. Stroke. 2006; 37(9):2331–2335

[417] Van Peppen RP, Kwakkel G, Wood-Dauphinee S, Hendriks HJ, Van der Wees PJ, Dekker J. The impact of physical therapy on functional outcomes after stroke: what's the evidence? Clin Rehabil. 2004; 18(8):833–862

[418] Vaney C, Roth R. Rehabilitation bei Multipler Sklerose (MS). In: Frommelt P, Lösslein H, Hrsg. NeuroRehabilitation. 3. Aufl. Heidelberg: Springer; 2010

[419] Velikonja O, Curić K, Ozura A, Jazbec SS. Influence of sports climbing and yoga on spasticity, cognitive function, mood and fatigue in patients with multiple sclerosis. Clin Neurol Neurosurg. 2010; 112(7):597–601

[420] Verschuren O, Ketelaar M, Takken T, Helders PJ, Gorter JW. Exercise programs for children with cerebral palsy: a systematic review of the literature. Am J Phys Med Rehabil. 2008; 87(5):404–417

[421] Viebrock H, Forst B. 2008

[422] Volpe BT, Krebs HI, Hogan N, Edelstein OTR L, Diels C, Aisen M. A novel approach to stroke rehabilitation: robot-aided sensorimotor stimulation. Neurology. 2000; 54(10):1938–1944

[423] von der Heyden S, Emons G, Viereck V. Hilgers R. Effect on muscles of mechanical vibrations produced by the Galileo 2000 in combination with physical therapy in treating female stress urinary incontinence. Proceedings of the Congress of International Continence Society 2003. Department of Gynecology and Obstetrics, 2003;s. 285

[424] Weimann G. Klinischer Einsatz der Krankengymnastik. In: Gutenbrunner C, Weimann G, Hrsg. Krankengymnastische Methoden und Konzepte. Heidelberg: Springer; 2004

[425] Weiss T, Miltner WHR. Motorisches Lernen – neuere Erkenntnisse und ihre Bedeutung für die motorische Rehabilitation. Z f (Zeitschrift Pflaum Verlag München) Physiotherapeuten. 2001; 53:578–588

[426] Weiss A, Suzuki T, Bean J, Fielding RA. High intensity strength training improves strength and functional performance after stroke. Am J Phys Med Rehabil. 2000; 79(4):369–376; quiz 391–394

[427] Wen CP, Wai JP, Tsai MK, et al. Minimum amount of physical activity for reduced mortality and extended life expectancy: a prospective cohort study. Lancet. 2011; 378(9798):1244–1253

[428] Wernig A, Müller S. Laufband locomotion with body weight support improved walking in persons with severe spinal cord injuries. Paraplegia. 1992; 30(4):229–238

[429] Whitall J, McCombe Waller S, Silver KH, Macko RF. Repetitive bilateral arm training with rhythmic auditory cueing improves motor function in chronic hemiparetic stroke. Stroke. 2000; 31(10):2390–2395

[430] White LJ, McCoy SC, Castellano V, et al. Resistance training improves strength and functional capacity in persons with multiple sclerosis. Mult Scler. 2004; 10(6):668–674

[431] Wicklein EM, Pfeiffer G, Ratusinski T, Kunze K. Type I Charcot-Marie-Tooth Syndrom. Disability and management [Article in German]. Nervenarzt. 1997; 68(4):358–362

[432] Wiesinger GF, Quittan M, Aringer M, et al. Improvement of physical fitness and muscle strength in polymyositis/dermatomyositis patients by a training programme. Br J Rheumatol. 1998a; 37(2):196–200

[433] Wiesinger GF, Quittan M, Graninger M, et al. Benefit of 6 months long-term physical training in polymyositis/dermatomyositis patients. Br J Rheumatol. 1998b; 37(12):1338–1342

[434] Willoughby KL, Dodd KJ, Shields N. A systematic review of the effectiveness of treadmill training for children with cerebral palsy. Disabil Rehabil. 2009; 31(24):1971–1979

[435] Winstein CJ, Rose DK, Tan SM, Lewthwaite R, Chui HC, Azen SP. A randomized controlled comparison of upper-extremity rehabilitation strategies in acute stroke: A pilot study of immediate and long-term outcomes. Arch Phys Med Rehabil. 2004; 85(4):620–628

[436] Winter S, Ludolph AC. Motoneuronerkrankungen. In: Winkler J, Ludolph A, Hrsg. Neurodegenerative Erkrankungen des Alters. Stuttgart: Thieme; 2004

[437] Woldag H, Hummelsheim H. Evidence-based physiotherapeutic concepts for improving arm and hand function in stroke patients: a review. J Neurol. 2002; 249(5):518–528

[438] Wolf PA, Cobb JL, D'Agostino RB. Epidemiology of stroke. In: Barnett HJM, Mohr JP, Stein BM, Yatsu FM, eds. Stroke: pathophysiology, diagnosis and management. New York: Churchill Livingston; 1992:3–27

[439] Wolf SL, Lecraw DE, Barton LA, Jann BB. Forced use of hemiplegic upper extremities to reverse the effect of learned nonuse among chronic stroke and head-injured patients. Exp Neurol. 1989; 104(2):125–132

[440] Wolf SL, Winstein CJ, Miller JP, et al; EXCITE Investigators. Effect of constraint-induced movement therapy on upper extremity function 3 to 9 months after stroke: the EXCITE randomized clinical trial. JAMA. 2006; 296(17):2095–2104

[441] Wolf SL, Winstein CJ, Miller JP, et al. Retention of upper limb function in stroke survivors who have received constraint-induced movement therapy: the EXCITE randomised trial. Lancet Neurol. 2008; 7(1):33–40

[442] Wolfsegger T, Stieglbauer K, Topakian R Weiss EM, Aichner FT. Belastungsintensitäten für ein Ausdauer- und

Krafttraining bei Patienten mit Myasthenia gravis. Dtsch Z Sportmed. 2011; 62(5):125–129

[443] Wright NC, Kilmer DD, McCrory MA, Aitkens SG, Holcomb BJ, Bernauer EM. Aerobic walking in slowly progressive neuromuscular disease: effect of a 12-week program. Arch Phys Med Rehabil. 1996; 77(1):64–69

[444] Wulf G. Motorisches Lernen: Einflussgröße und ihrer Optimierung. In: Dettmers Ch, Bülau P, Weiller C, Hrsg. Schlaganfall Rehabilitation. Bad Honnef:Hippocampus; 2007

[445] Wulf G, Clauss A, Shea CH, Whitacre CA. Benefits of self-control in dyad practice. Res Q Exerc Sport. 2001; 72(3):299–303

[446] Wulf G, McConnel N, Gärtner M, Schwarz A. Enhancing the learning of sport skills through external-focus feedback. J Mot Behav. 2002; 34(2):171–182

[447] Wulf G, Raupach M, Pfeiffer F. Self-controlled observational practice enhances learning. Res Q Exerc Sport. 2005; 76(1):107–111

[448] Wulf G, Shea CH. Understanding the role of augmented feedback: the good, the bad and the ugly. In: Williams A, Hodges NJ, eds. Skil acquisition in sport:Research, theory and practice. London: Routlede; 2004:121–144

[449] Wulf G, Toole T. Physical assistance devices in complex motor skill learning: benefits of a self-controlled practice schedule. Res Q Exerc Sport. 1999; 70(3):265–272

[450] Yang YR, Wang RY, Lin KH, Chu MY, Chan RC. Task-oriented progressive resistance strength training improves muscle strength and functional performance in individuals with stroke. Clin Rehabil. 2006; 20(10):860–870

[451] Zäch G, Koch HG. Paraplegie. Ganzheitliche Rehabilitation. Freiburg: Karger; 2006

[452] Zerres K, Rudnik-Schöneborn S, Wirth B. Proximale spinale Muskelatrophien. Dtsch Arztebl. 1998; 95(26):A-1667–A-1674

[453] Ziegler K. Evidenzbasierte Physiotherapie bei Multipler Sklerose. Nervenheilkunde. 2007; 12:1088–1094

[454] Zierz S, Jerusalem F. Muskelerkrankungen: Referenz-Reihe Neurologie. 3. Aufl. Stuttgart: Thieme; 2003

[455] Zwecker M, Zeilig G, Ohry A. Professor Heinrich Sebastian Frenkel: a forgotten founder of rehabilitation medicine. Spinal Cord. 2004; 42(1):55–56

[456] Zwick H, ed. Bewegung als Therapie: gezielte Schritte zum Wohlbefinden. 2. Aufl. Heidelberg: Springer; 2006

Index

A

Action Research Arm Test (ARAT) 98, 101, 102, 103
acute inflammatory demyelinating polyradiculoneuropathy 92
Amadeo Rehabilitation robot 26
amyotrophic lateral sclerosis 90
anterior horn cell disorders 90
arm ability, basis training 108. See also impairment-oriented training
Armeo Power robot 26
Armeo Spring robot 26, 27
Ashworth scale, spasticity 35, 36
assessments and tests 98, 108. See also specific tools
ataxia
– cycling trainers 57
– SpaceCurl 66, 67
– symptoms of 38, 39, 40
Austrian Mobility Scale (AMS) 101, 102, 103

B

balance
– Berg Balance Scale (BBS) 101, 102, 103, 104
– MTD device 68, 70
– pads 67
– Parkinson's disease 84
– Physiomat 67
– Posturomed 67, 68
– Sensamove 69
– SpaceCurl 65, 66, 67
– symptoms of 40, 41
– Terrasensa 67, 68, 69
– trainers 64, 65, 66
– training in 16, 40, 41, 63
– treadmill training 49, 50
Barthel Index 101, 102, 103
Becker muscular dystrophy 93
Berg Balance Scale (BBS) 101, 102, 103, 104
bilateral training principles 24, 25, 26
Bi-Manu-Track 24, 25
Borg scale 80
boulder walls 72
Box and Block Test (BBT) 98, 101, 102, 103
butterfly reverse 61

C

cardiovascular rehabilitation 4, 10
cerebral palsy 87
Charcot, Jean-Marie 69
Charcot–Marie–Tooth disease 91

CIMT

CIMT 108. See also constraint-induced movement therapy
climbing 71
climbing walls 61, 72, 77, 78
clinical pictures 108. See also see specific conditions
congenital myopathies 94
constraint-induced movement therapy
– efficacy of 21
– learned non-use 21, 22, 23
– lower extremity 22
– principles of 21
– upper vs. lower extremity 21, 22
craniocerebral trauma 86
critical illness myopathy 92
critical illness polyneuropathy 92
cycle ergometers 53
cycling trainers 35
– arm paresis accessories 56
– ataxia patients 57
– duration of training 58
– foot binding 56
– forms of training 57, 58
– hemiparesis patients 58
– overview 55, 56
– pain management 57
– Parkinson's disease 58
– spasticity and 57, 58
– stroke patients 58
– symmetrical training 55, 56
– training controlled by power output 54
– with feedback 56, 57

D

deconditioning syndrome 11, 86
Duchenne muscular dystrophy 93
Dynamic Gait Index (DGI) 98, 101, 102, 103

E

elliptical trainers 54, 55
endurance
– cycling trainers 108
– elliptical trainers 54, 55
– leg presses 60
– neuromuscular disorders 89
– paraplegic patients 86
– Parkinson's disease 85
– steppers 58, 59
– stroke patients 77, 78
– training controlled by power output 54
– training equipment 42
– treadmill training 48, 49, 101, 102, 103
– upper body ergometers 53, 54
ergometer training 4
Erigo 28, 29, 59, 77

EX90

EX90 elliptical trainer 54, 55
Expanded Disability Status Scale (EDSS) 101, 102, 103, 104, 105

F

facilities 97
feedback training
– acoustic 30
– principles of 30
– verbal 30
– vestibular 30, 31
– visual 30, 31
fever disorders 70
Foerster, Otfrid 2
Frankfurt Institute for Brain Trauma Patients 3
Freezing of Gait Questionnaire (FOGQ) 101, 102, 103, 105, 106
Frenkel, Heinrich S. 2
Fugl–Meyer Test (FM) 101, 102, 103
Functional Ambulation Categories (FAC) 101, 102, 103, 106
Functional Independence Measure (FIM) 101, 102, 103, 106, 107
Functional Reach Test (FRT) 99, 101, 102, 103

G

Gelb, Adrémar 3
G-EO System Evolution 58, 59
German Association for Rehabilitation 2
GIGER MD 76, 77
Glasgow Coma Scale (GCS) 101, 102, 103
Goldstein, Kurt 3
Gross Motor Function Classification System (GMFCS) 101, 102, 103
Guillain–Barré syndrome 92
Guttmann, Ludwig 85

H

HapticWalker 58, 59
heel-to-knee test 40
hereditary neuropathy 91
hereditary spastic paraplegia 95
Hoehn–Yahr scale 82
Holten, Oddvar 4
Höppner, Heidi 17

I

ICF biopsychosocial model 17, 18
impairment-oriented training principles 23

K

knee extension training, leg presses 60, 61
Kugelberg-Welander disease 91

L

Lambert–Eaton myasthenic syndrome 93
lat-pull machines 61, 62, 78
learned non-use 21, 22, 23
leg curl machine 63, 64
leg presses 60, 61
limb–girdle muscular dystrophies 94
Ling, Pehr Henrik 1
LokoHelp 26, 28, 44
LokoHelp Pedago 45
Lokomat 27, 28, 44, 52, 76
long barbells 62, 64

M

Medical Research Council Scale (MRC) 101, 102, 103
Mirror Image Movement Enabler (MIME) robot 25
mirror therapy principles 29, 30
MIT Manus 25
modified Karvonen's formula 52
mononeuropathy 91
MoreGait 27, 29
MOTOmed Letto 2 76
motor learning
– factors affecting 32
– feedback, positive 33
– pauses, planned 33
– randomized practice 33
– repetition in 33
– training, dosage 33
– training effects 11, 18
– training, organization of 33
– variability in 34
motor neuron disorders 90
motor rehabilitation 19, 20
movement
– chronic diseases and 8
– decreased exercise tolerance 11
– inactivity, consequences of 9, 11
– inflammatory substances induction by 7, 8
– interleukin-1 (IL-1) induction by 7
– interleukin-6 (IL-6) induction by 7
– locomotion, recommendations 8, 9
– myokines and 8
– positive effects of 9, 10
– significance of 6, 7
– studies of 7, 8
– tumor necrosis factor alpha (TNF-α) induction by 7

MTD device **68**, *70*
multiple sclerosis
– Borg scale 80
– dorsiflexion training 78
– fatigue, exhaustion in 79
– outcomes 81
– pauses, planned 79, 80
– severely impaired patients 81
– training principles 80
– training recommendations 79, 80
– treadmill training 79
– Uhthoff phenomenon 79
– upper motor neuron syndrome 78
– WEIMuS *101*, *102*, *103*, 107
muscular dystrophy **93**
muscular strength scale (MRC) 11
myasthenia gravis **93**
myositis **94**

N

neuromuscular disorders 108
– classification of *89*
– endurance training recommendations **89**
– general notes **88**
– ion channel disorders **94**
– metabolic myopathies **94**
– motor neuron disorders **90**
– myopathies **93**
– overview 88
– strength training recommendations **89**
– toxic myopathies **95**
neuropathy **91**
neurorehabilitation 108
– arm stretches **14**, *15*, *16*
– coordination training in **16**
– cortical reorganization **17**
– elasticity, joint mobility in **14**, *15*
– endurance training in **13**
– evidence, hierarchy of *17*, *18*
– ICF biopsychosocial model *17*, *18*
– learning, forms of *18*, *19*
– leg stretches **14**, *15*
– social group effect *19*
– speed training in **13**
– strength training in **12**
– transfer problem 19, *20*
Nine Hole Peg Test (NHPT) *99*, *101*, *102*, *103*
NuStep elliptical trainer 54, *55*

O

Oskar Helene Home 2

P

Pablo system 26, *27*
paraplegia *85*, *86*, *87*
Parkinson's disease
– balance training 84
– cognitive motion strategies 85

– cycling trainers 58, 82
– endurance training in 85
– home exercises for *85*
– mobile stability training 83
– motor rehabilitation focus 81, 82
– postural stability training 83
– prevalence of 81
– strength training in 82, 83, 85
– therapeutic exercise in 32
– training goals 81, *82*
– treadmill training in 47, 82, 85
– Unified Parkinson's Disease Rating Scale (UPDRS) *101*, *102*, *103*
– vibration training 82
Performance Oriented Mobility Assessment (POMA) *101*, *102*, *103*
peripheral neuropathy **92**
personnel requirements **97**
Physiomat **67**
Pintsch, Oskar and Helene 2
post polio syndrome **91**
postural control 108
Posturomed **67**, *68*
Power Plate **71**
Prussian Cripple Care Act of 1920 2
pusher syndrome 66, *67*

R

Reha-Digit 25, *26*
Reha-Slide 25
Reha-Slide-Duo 25
repetitive sensorimotor hand training principles **23**
Rivermead ADL scale *101*, *102*, *103*
Rivermead Mobility Index *101*, *102*, *103*
robot-assisted training
– gait trainers 26, *27*, *28*, *29*
– principles **25**, *26*, *27*
– treadmill training 108
Robowalk 26, *28*
Romberg test *40*

S

Sanatorium Schloss Rheinburg 3
Sandow, Eugene (Friedrich Wilhelm Müller) 3
Schmieder, Friedrich 3
Schütz, Hans 2
Schwarzenegger, Arnold 3
Sensamove **69**
SilverFit **72**
slacklining **72**
SpaceCurl **65**, *66*, *67*
spasticity
– clonus test 36, *37*
– cycling trainers 35, 57, 58
– findings in **35**, *36*, *37*
– in stroke patients 74
– post-stroke 34
– severity of 35, *36*, *37*
– symptoms of **35**

– treadmill training **51**
– walking training 35, *36*
speed
– training effects **13**
– training in neurorehabilitation **13**
– treadmill training **50**, *51*, *101*, *102*, *103*
speed-dependent treadmill training **50**, *101*, *102*, *103*, 108
spinal muscular atrophy **90**
SRT/Zeptor **70**
strength, strength training
– butterfly reverse **61**
– climbing walls **61**, *72*
– effects of **11**, 59
– in neurologic patients, parameters *60*
– in Parkinson's disease 82, 83, 85
– knee extensors, flexors **63**, *64*
– lat-pull machines **61**, *62*, *78*
– leg curl machine 63, *64*
– leg presses **60**, *61*
– long barbells 62, *64*
– neuromuscular disorders **89**
– principles of **24**
– short barbells *62*
– stroke patients 74, **77**
– treadmill training **49**, *50*
– weight bars *62*, *63*
Stroke Impact Scale (SIS) *101*, *102*, *103*, 108
stroke patients 74
– aerobic training guidelines 76
– climbing walls 77, *78*
– cycling trainers 58
– disability extent, severity 73
– early mobilization, rehabilitation 76, *77*
– endurance **77**, *78*
– epidemiology 73
– motion pattern, preferred 74
– motor skills evaluation 74
– outcomes 76
– oxygen intake, maximum 73
– postural control 76
– SpaceCurl 66
– spasticity and 74
– strength training 74, **77**
– therapeutic exercise benefits 73
– therapeutic exercise recommendations **75**
– treadmill training 75, *76*
– upper motor neuron syndrome 74

T

Tardieu scale, spasticity 36, *37*
target heart rate (THR) 52
Terrasensa **67**, *68*, *69*
tests and assessments 98, 108
therapeutic exercise 108
– benefits of 32

– clinical applications of 4, *5*
– cripple care programs 2
– development as specialty **3**, *4*
– early history of 1, 2
– facilities required for **97**
– Nazi period 3
– personnel requirements **97**
– post-WWII 3
– Schmieder's principles 3
– severely impaired patients **95**
– shaping, adoption of 2
– training, planning of **96**
– treadmill therapy 108
– treatable neurologic symptoms in **34**
– WWI 3
Timed "Up and Go" (TUG) *101*, *102*, *103*
Time Walking Test *101*, *102*, *103*
Tinetti Score *101*, *102*, *103*
Tissot, Joseph Clément 1
training effects
– balance **16**
– coordination **16**
– endurance **13**
– foot dorsiflexors 12
– gait improvement 13
– hip flexors 12
– mobility **14**
– motor skills, basic **11**, 18
– muscular endurance, power 12
– plantar flexors 12
– plasticity **17**
– quadriceps 12
– speed **13**
– strength, strength skills **11**
training equipment **42**
transfer problem 19, *20*
treadmill training
– advantages of 46, *47*
– balance **49**, *50*
– body weight–supported *43*
– central pattern generators (CPGs) 44, *46*
– cerebral palsy 87
– clinical applications 47
– dual-task, multi-task 46, **50**
– endurance 48, *101*, *102*, *103*
– endurance training **49**
– equipment **42**, *43*, *44*
– gait trainers 43, *44*
– HR$_{max}$ 52
– in Parkinson's disease 82, 85
– long barbells 62, *64*
– multiple sclerosis 79
– patient's feet, advancing 52
– principles of 4, *5*, 27
– public transportation, escalators 48
– slat-belt treadmill *43*, *44*
– spasticity **51**
– speed **50**, *51*, *101*, *102*, *103*
– strength **49**, *50*
– strength training 49
– stride reaction reinforcement 47
– stroke patients 75, *76*
– target heart rate (THR) 52
– training intensity 52

- training intensity, β-blockers 52
- walking backward on 52
- walking, efficient 47
- walking, minimum speeds 47
- walking motion sequence 44, 46
- walking outside home 48
- weight bars 62, 63, 64
- with forearm supports 43

U

Unified Parkinson's Disease Rating Scale (UPDRS) 101, 102, 103

Unterberger test 40
upper body ergometers 53, 54
upper motor neuron syndrome 74, 78
- ataxia 38, 40, 108
- balance, postural control 40, 41
- paresis 36, 38
- spasticity 108
- symptoms 34

V

vibration training
- climbing 71
- contraindications 70
- effects of 69, 71
- Galileo 71
- Galileo vs. vertical, effects of 71
- overview 69
- Parkinson's disease 82
- Power Plate 71
- SRT/Zeptor 70
- Wellengang 71
virtual reality training principles 29

W

weight bars 62, 63
Werdnig–Hoffmann disease 90
whole body vibration (WBV) 108
Wolf Motor Function Test 99, 101, 102, 103
Würzburg Fatigue Inventory for MS (WEIMuS) 101, 102, 103, 107

Y

YouGrabber 26, 27

Z

Zander, Gustav 1